Antonina Kravtsova

How the world speaks with us

Use of Grigori Grabovoi's technologies in everyday life

2017

How the world speaks with us. Use of Grigori Grabovoi's technologies in everyday life

Derivative work was written on the basis of materials of the Teachings of Grigori Grabovoi. You will find a lot of interesting and useful information. Get acquainted with the materials, testimonies, articles. Material gives awareness to realize the level of macro salvation and to apply it actively for solution of your own objectives. It is based on the perception of Grigori Grabovoi's technologies in relation to the person, because in the technogenic world it is difficult to apply to oneself technological understanding of the normalization of events and health, although the foundations of the Divine development of the world are laid in methods.

Jelezky Publishing, Hamburg

www.jelezky-publishing.com

1. Edition, май 2017. - 56 p.

© 2017, Jelezky publishing UG (Publisher), Hamburg

SVET UG, Hamburg

2017-1, 10.05.2017

ISBN: 978-3-945549-36-0
© Кравцова Антонина, 2017

CONTENT

Level of Beauty and Eternity
of the Teaching of Grigori Grabovoi

Watching the photos of the nature of Earth has often caused such associations that I would like to describe my understanding of the level of highness and beauty in the Teachings of Grigori Grabovoi.

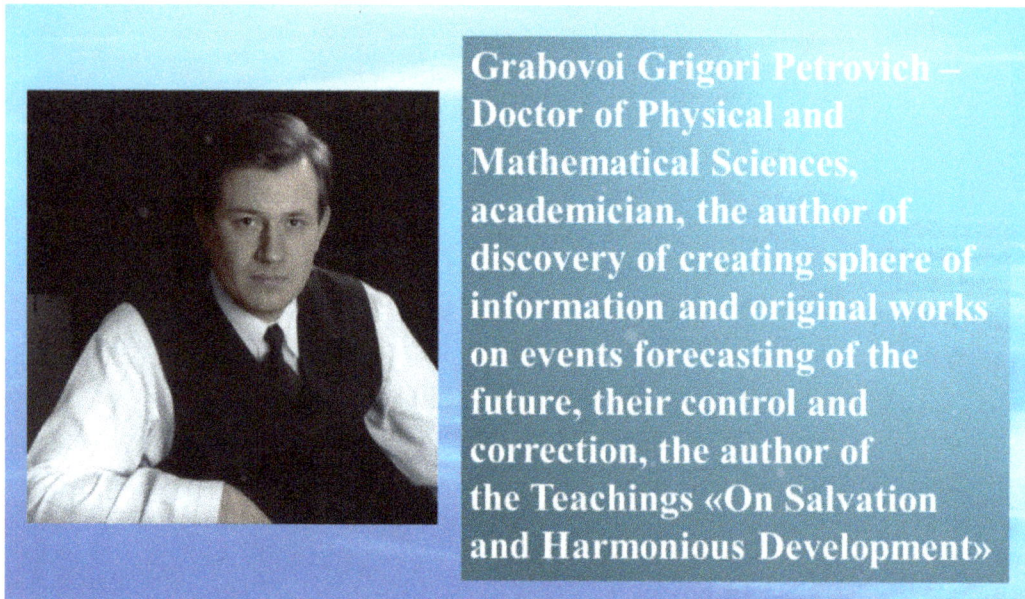

Grabovoi Grigori Petrovich – Doctor of Physical and Mathematical Sciences, academician, the author of discovery of creating sphere of information and original works on events forecasting of the future, their control and correction, the author of the Teachings «On Salvation and Harmonious Development»

The beauty of nature gives a thrill, specially with a man standing on the top.

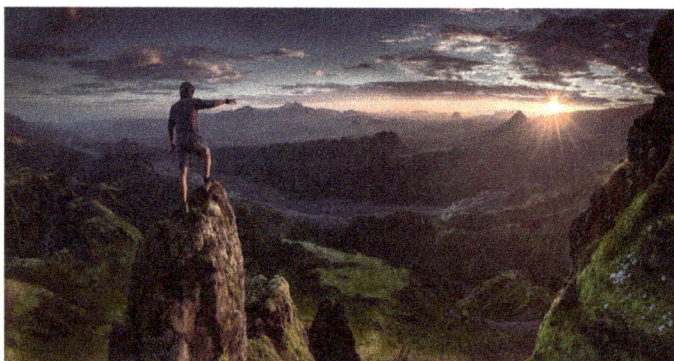

Man climbs to the top of understanding and begins to see the world quite differently when starting to learn, to know, to perceive the Teaching through the interest, which he may experience like it is shown in the films about nature, for example, through the beauty of nature and delight. That is just like when, firstly, man enjoys climbing up, he is aware that Divine beauty and insight would reveal for him and that would be understanding of Knowledge.

And there's more – that's not the ultimate dream. Then infinity of space and eternity of the world open, that's what is in the film. So, man can develop himself so much with the help of technologies of the Teachings up to the level that he would be able to see everything and by himself at once: his personality (the Soul, Spirit, Consciousness, physical body) perceives himself in any event, as if from outside, that is a higher level, while controlling external events to the smallest detail.

So then man makes only the correct and harmonious steps, because man follows in the footsteps of God.

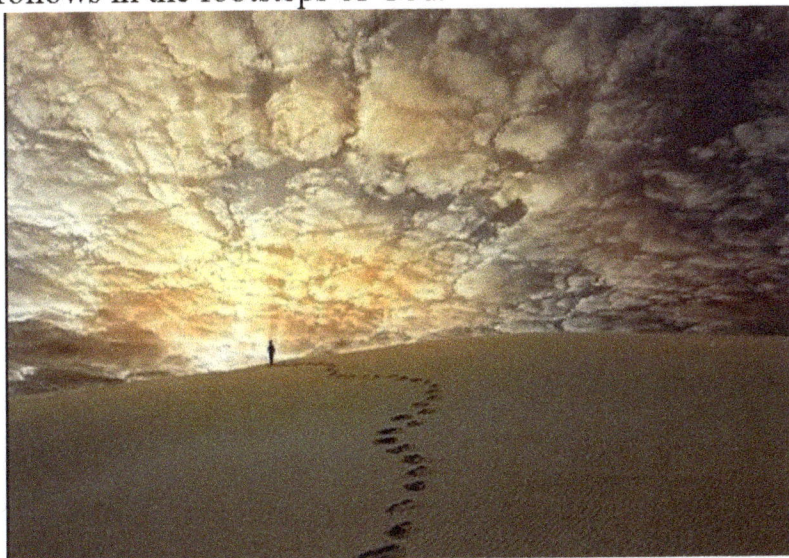

That is the **Beauty of the Teachings of Grigori Grabovoi.**
October 7th, 2016.

Recovery of Computer Control System

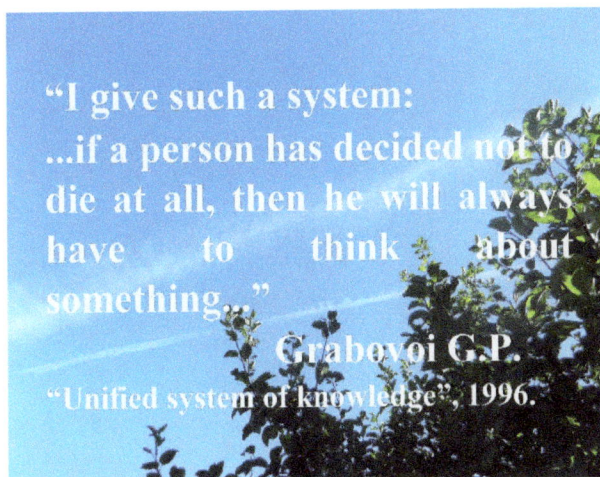

"I give such a system: ...if a person has decided not to die at all, then he will always have to think about something..."

Grabovoi G.P.
"Unified system of knowledge", 1996.

The 31 August 2016 when viewing files on the old computer once again there happened crashing programs and files stopped to open, the off button didn't work and so on (that`s why, in principle, the new computer was bought, but almost the whole archive remained in the old computer).

The 1 September it was decided to transfer basic information to the new computer via the upload on the flash drive. Files didn`t still open, video was impossible to watch, it was possible just to download, and on the other computer all perfectly replicated.

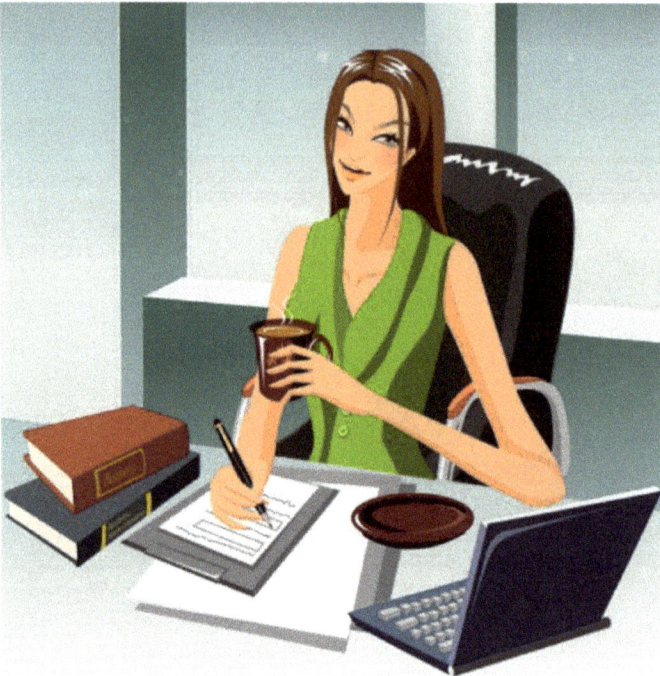

And suddenly the light was turned off, the computer was incorrectly shut down, although before too there were cases when it was necessary to turn off the system by means of power method: Ctrl+Alt+Delete.

After a 15 minute break, I turned on the computer and after some time saw that the updates are almost downloaded.

It is at this moment I applied the equation from the theory of generalized functions.

$$g = (f(k(I)) * f(k(P)))^{x^n}$$

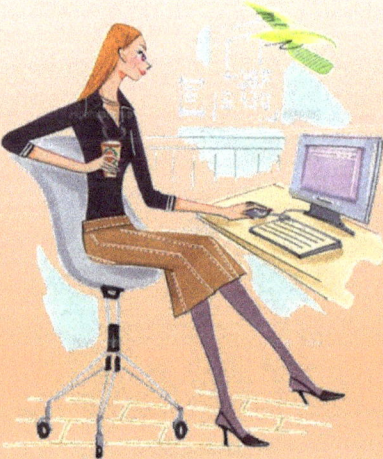

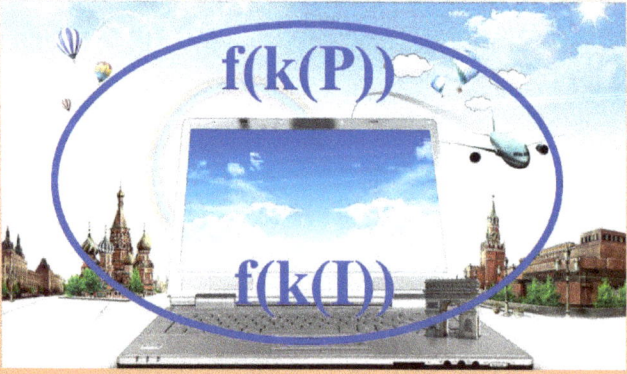

How did I watch? I watched external space from where the updates are downloaded, saw the border of information downloading and kept the internal computer circuit in the norm.

The Equation from the Theory of Generalized Functions

$$g = (f(k(I)) * f(k(P)))^{x^n}$$

g – the generalized function;
$f(k(I))$ – the individual function;
$f(k(P))$ – the function from the space;
X^n – the degree expresses the law of changes of common connections. The taking decision depends on X^n.

The coordinates of the process or events are defined in the parameter X – it is approximately or exactly. You need to change the process to the direction of this possible catastrophe did not happen, doing concentration on X^n.

And mentally I saw the equation on the slide, where the whole process of technological application of this method is described (just remembered the slide).

The Equation from the Theory of Generalized Functions

The first level is the boundary between perception and reality

The second level – the connection between reality and your perception is summarized by a system of common connections.

$f(k(I))$ 1,2 $f(k(P))$

1   2

$$g = (f(k(I)) * f(k(P)))^{x^n}$$

g – the generalized function;
$f(k(I))$ – the individual function;
$f(k(P))$ – the function from the space;
X^n – the degree expresses the law of changes of common connections. The taking decision depends on X^n.

If you consider any element of reality, which is located at the junction between these two elements, then the generalized function g must contain, obviously, in the form of implicit area immediately the two positions.

The coordinates of the process or events are defined in the parameter X – it is approximately or exactly. You need to change the process to the direction of this possible catastrophe did not happen, doing concentration on X^n.

Further, as in the case of the refrigerator restoration, there was applied the method of normalization through sound. First there heard just some kind of grinding sound inside and out, but in order not to delay this process of listening, I quickly turned the grinding sound upon classical music – just heard a violin. Then I moved away from the computer so that the update process was normally ended.

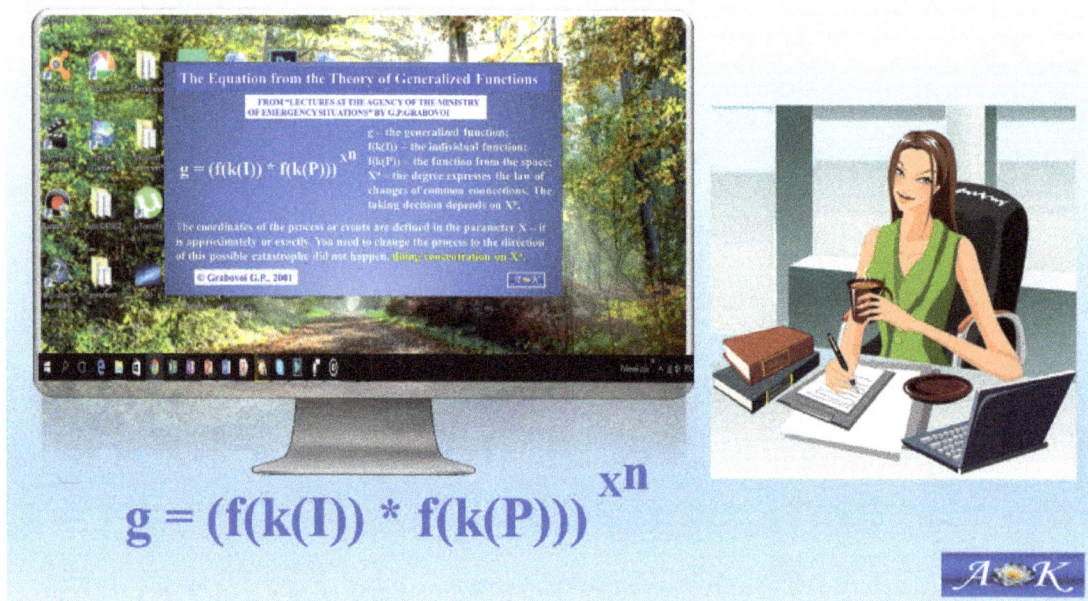

$$g = (f(k(I)) * f(k(P)))^{x^n}$$

Returning to the computer, the first thing I saw, was the normal operating line of the "basement" with all the icons that had disappeared at the time of failure. And then – all the files safely open, video and audio function... Computer is running again. I had the same cases before as well, and I used to work with the computer through the recovery point of computer control system. But this time I wasn't able to find this point, because nothing could be open, except for one file on the desktop (through which I worked).

This control, of course, was done in the level of already obtained result by somebody – the restoration of the refrigerator, repairing of the phone. If someone did this once, so it can be repeated many times.

This is not an introduction to higher mathematics, it is a simple and accurate control through concentration on the equation of G. P. Grabovoi.

Each person may have his/her own refinements and details of carrying out of control: you can add the sound to view the process normalizing, someone can probably see by direct vision, someone sees through color, and so on. It is a creative process. Thanks to Grigori Petrovich for the Knowledge HE gives.

September 2, 2016.

Oxygen Increasing in the Room According to the Teachings of Grigori Grabovoi

"...namely trying to understand, that is an introduction to the sphere of thinking, right?.. an increasing amount of information allows you to make material system. So how to obtain oxygen or to improve, for example, the oxygen in the room?

Oxygen increasing in the room according to the Teachings of Grigori Grabovoi

Volume of information

We need to collect as much information as possible around there - fifty hectares, for example, a three-kilometer height - and just squeeze.

An introduction to the sphere of thinking

© Grabovoi G.P., 2005

We need to collect as much information as possible around there – fifty hectares, right?.. for example, to take it volumetric, great, a three-kilometer height – and just squeeze, for example. Oxygen will be really increased. It is even possible to do it, when it is necessary for premises".

(Grigori Grabovoi, January 28, 2005)

Technology of Rejuvenating by the Book of Grigori Grabovoi "Number Series of Psychological Normalization"

This time I tried to choose a different couple of psychological terms, which could be at once clearer for many readers. It was decided to make the number series not very long, so they could be seen at the controlling scheme. As it is seen from the below technology, the number series should be located closely. That's important.

Technology:
6. The process of rejuvenating is carried out the following way:
6.1. Visualize that digits corresponding to one term are located from the shoulder to the wrist of the right hand.
6.2. Visualize that digits corresponding to the term, which follows the term described in the item 6.1 are located on the skin of the left hand.
6.3. Feel how light flows from the digits on the left hand to the digits on the right hand. During the period of this light flowing through the area of your chest, perceive how you have solved the psychological aspect of eternal development personally for yourself, as well as for all people around.

It is clear that you can take any pairs of number sequences when practicing this book. In my point of view, you can do it when you have practiced the technology precisely. Indeed, a lot of things are important: the number sequence located on the right hand is the first one, and the light from the left hand comes back to right hand being reflected from the second number sequence, which follows the first one. That's how information "flows" in the Author's book, and we go step by step from one term to another term.

So the number sequences are as follows.

For example, the number sequence **498714816** is located **on the right hand from the shoulder to the wrist**.

SUSCEPTIBILITY 498714816 – *the ability to have representations of different brightness and connection with the outside world, with varying degrees of feelings intensity. This quality of personality is derived from representations.*

That is important for me to realize the meaning of the number sequence, that is why I like the fact that **susceptibility** is *the ability to have representations of different brightness and connection with the outside world.* I allocate this number series as the first one on the right hand, and then write the number series on **the skin of the left hand**: **598712488212**.

As the skin is a boundary between the internal and external, then the term **susceptibility** is connected with the second term, which is linked with the outside world through hand skin.

The second term:

WARMING-UP – 598712488212 – *the process of adaptation to the actually performed activities, during which there is a setting of all psycho-physiological functions at the expense of actualization the dynamic stereotype. Herewith, there is an increase in neural irritability and functional mobility of the nervous system, with the increasing concentration of excitation of the nerve processes. This setting reduces the execution time of operations, improves the* *pace of work and its efficiency. Warming-up is usually complete within the first hour, followed by a steady operating state.*

And since then there is warming-up, a process of adaptation of the performed activity for **rejuvenation**, which goes through the number series and from the skin surface, from relations with the outside world. That's how the process of adaptation to the whole body occurs.

You read carefully the definition of **WARMING–UP**, and get aware how the whole process of *the nervous system* setting occurs. The numbers on the left hand do not exist in themselves, and they carry out the whole process of concentration of *excitation of nervous processes* **for rejuvenating the entire body** during the transmission of light through the chest. In the process of **rejuvenating**, feel firstly, then perceive *how you have solved the psychological aspect of eternal development personally for yourself, as well as for all people around.*

Solution of the psychological aspect of eternal development personally for yourself, as well as for all people around you

SUSCEPTIBILITY 498714816

WARMING–UP 598712488212

© Grabovoi G.P., 2003

And the process results that the light from the number series on the skin of the left hand is connected with the number series on the right hand.

This means that warming-up – or the process of adaptation... – leads in this case to *the ability to have representations of different brightness and connection with the outside world.*

Technology of Rejuvenating by the Book of G.P. Grabovoi "Number Series of Psychological Normalization"

SUSCEPTIBILITY 498714816 – the ability to have representations of different brightness and connection with the outside world...

WARMING-UP – 598712488212 – the process of adaptation to the actually performed activities...

4 9 8 7 1 4 8 1 6

598712488212

Technology:

6. The process of rejuvenating is carried out the following way:

6.1. Visualize that digits corresponding to one term are located from the shoulder to the wrist of the right hand.

6.2. Visualize that digits corresponding to the term, which follows the term described in the item 6.1 are located on the skin of the left hand.

6.3. Feel how light flows from the digits on the left hand to the digits on the right hand. During the period of this light flowing through the area of your chest, perceive how you have solved the psychological aspect of eternal development personally for yourself, as well as for all people around.

© Grabovoi G.P., 2003

In the process of rejuvenating we perceive the **aspect of eternal development.** It means that we rejuvenate for ETERNAL DEVELOPMENT, and not to have a beautiful body just right now, though – and for that, too. This is a mandatory goal – **ETERNAL DEVELOPMENT.** And development happens at once during the rejuvenation process. For example, the term **susceptibility** also includes the "quality of personality, which is derived from representations."

While working with this number sequence, we're working with it at the time of control: we normalize **susceptibility**, and acquire the ability to have representations. This is important in technological processes. When working with the second sequence, we learn the process of adaptation, i.e. warming-up, getting into a steady operating state.

It turns out that we actually work with two terms, normalizing our abilities, while simultaneously visualizing number series in the right place. And the way of imagining numerical rows and the transmission of light through the chest is a technology of rejuvenating. As you can see, there is a multi-level control, where *the aspect of eternal development* is an important part in the work with both terms and a technology of rejuvenating. People must be aware of their eternity.

From the above reasoning it is clear that it is important to choose a couple of psychological terms appropriately for this technology of rejuvenating. In the shown example, *setting* **for warming-up** *reduces the execution time of operations.*

Rejuvenation for Women and Men

Material from the interview of Grigori Grabovoi given to the reporter of the magazine "SOBESEDNIK".

It is possible to maintain own physical body in the state of normal health and youth using the technologies which are described in the works of doctor of physico-mathematical Sciences Grigori Petrovich Grabovoi.

Interesting technologies, including technologies of rejuvenation were given by Grigori Grabovoi in his interview to the reporter of the magazine **"SOBESEDNIK"**, October 4, 2005.

Humanity on the path of its evolutionary development takes into account, of course, different directions: of course, such disruptive technologies to save people from serious diseases through rejuvenation according to clinical scores are important.

Technologies concern radical life extension and the return of youth to the structures of physical body.

You can listen to a fragment of the interview of Grigori Petrovich Grabovoi in video material.

Fragment from the interview of Grigori Petrovich Grabovoi, of October 4, 2005:

Grabovoi G. P. – Yes, I just put the thoughts in the right spot. For example, to rejuvenate the woman according to clinical – well, that is if there are other diseases – it`s necessary to focus in the area of the left elbow. I have the technologies, they are described. If just to rejuvenate, it's right elbow, and so on. That is, in fact, it is a technology.

Reporter - to look there, right? And to think, right?.. about something?
Grabovoi G. P. – Yes, to concentrate and to see, to imagine, say, the glow of silvery light, – and that`s all – around 5 minutes. But it is for women. There is another technology for men.
Reporter – Really?
Grabovoi G. P. – Yes. Male rejuvenation is a left heel, a little higher. And then the knee joint from the inside. And, therefore, prevention, well, that is if there are problems...

But, as a rule, it`s enough for men to apply rejuvenation without emphasis on the disease. It`s easier for men, - just men are healthy, right?.. In principle. Version. If, nevertheless, there is the emphasis, then – if the person is considered to be sickly – then it's all the same the right knee joint, but the front part.

By the way, people work very efficiently, a lot of academics I know, just concentrate and actually feel the skin beginning to stretch. That is, they rejuvenate, do medical tests. Then they compare tests – the tests are such as, for example, minus 20 years – blood tests, there and so on.

In the end of the interview Grigori Petrovich tells:

"Well, actually, you know, I think that everyone should be able to – well, treat one another, right? from any disease, not necessarily from, well AIDS. Therefore, in principle, in my opinion, the situation is such that you just have to work as much as possible and that`s all."

But what is remarkable in this interview is that the reporter probably would like to have someone doing the same job, for example, at least for rejuvenation. So he calmly suggests: *"It will be like to go to the manicurist now, right? In general, one had a wish and went".*

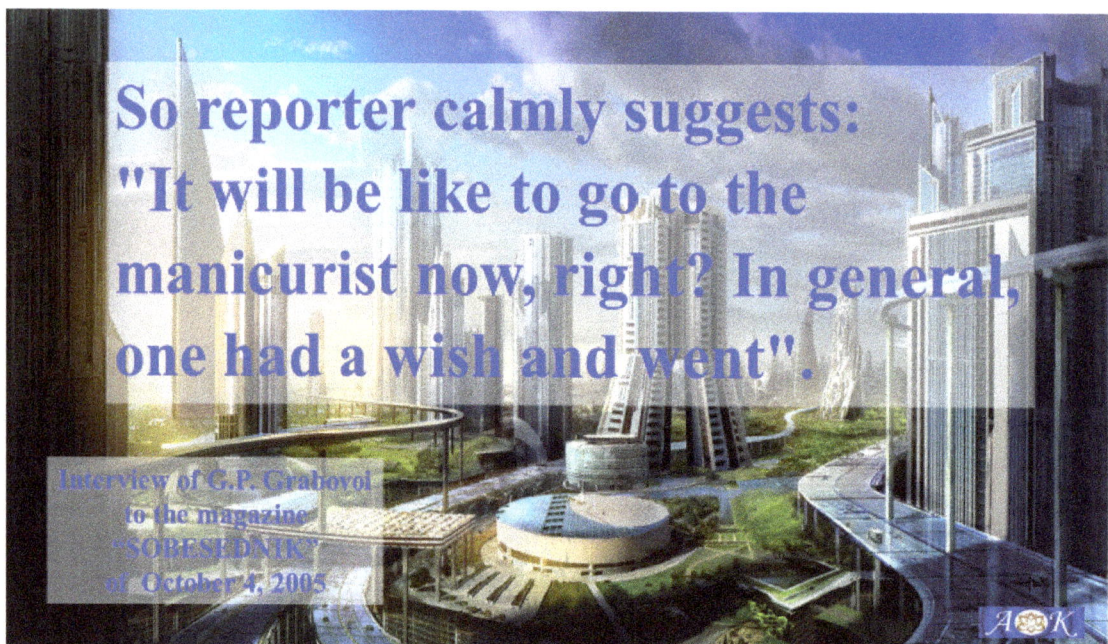

So reporter calmly suggests:
"It will be like to go to the manicurist now, right? In general, one had a wish and went".

Interview of G.P. Graboyoi
to the magazine
"SOBESEDNIK"
of October 4, 2005

And Grigori Petrovich Grabovoi replies: *"Not exactly, but approximately. In around two hundred and fifty years there will be such a technology available – very fast, but until then this technology will be slow. Well, maybe. Although civilization can begin to develop – we're all controllers. And then the*

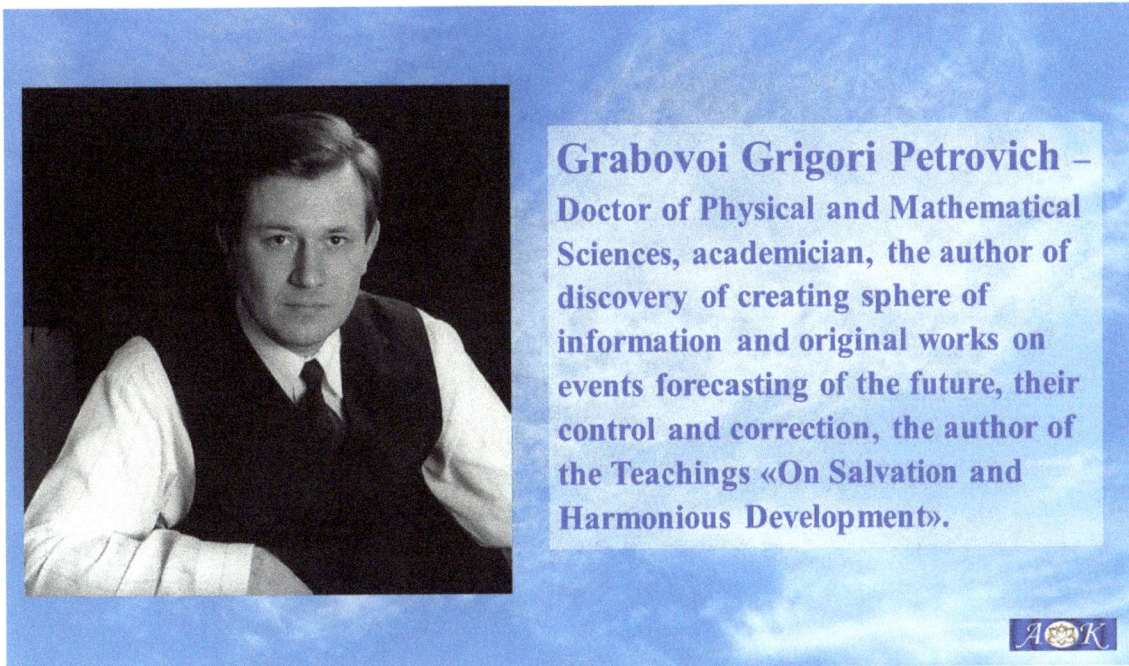

Grabovoi Grigori Petrovich – Doctor of Physical and Mathematical Sciences, academician, the author of discovery of creating sphere of information and original works on events forecasting of the future, their control and correction, the author of the Teachings «On Salvation and Harmonious Development».

person can rejuvenate faster, in a short time – it is possible".

This answer, firstly, gives hope and confidence that we will live to see that time, because everything is acquired by practice: it means that the rapid rejuvenation technologies will come after slow ones. Secondly, this current time we will rejuvenate slowly if we don't want all together to do it quickly. It turns out that civilization may begin to develop very quickly.

And thirdly, in the book by Grigori Grabovoi "Hayrúkulus" it is written so:
«Thus, Hayrúkulus saw the evolution of the people in themselves, when everyone can develop as much as he wants. At that what is outside, it will flow in to him as much as he needs. Thus, Hayrúkulus saw the golden age of humanity and of the whole world, and he realized that this century will never be over. Other civilizations began to flock to this light that flared up more and more».

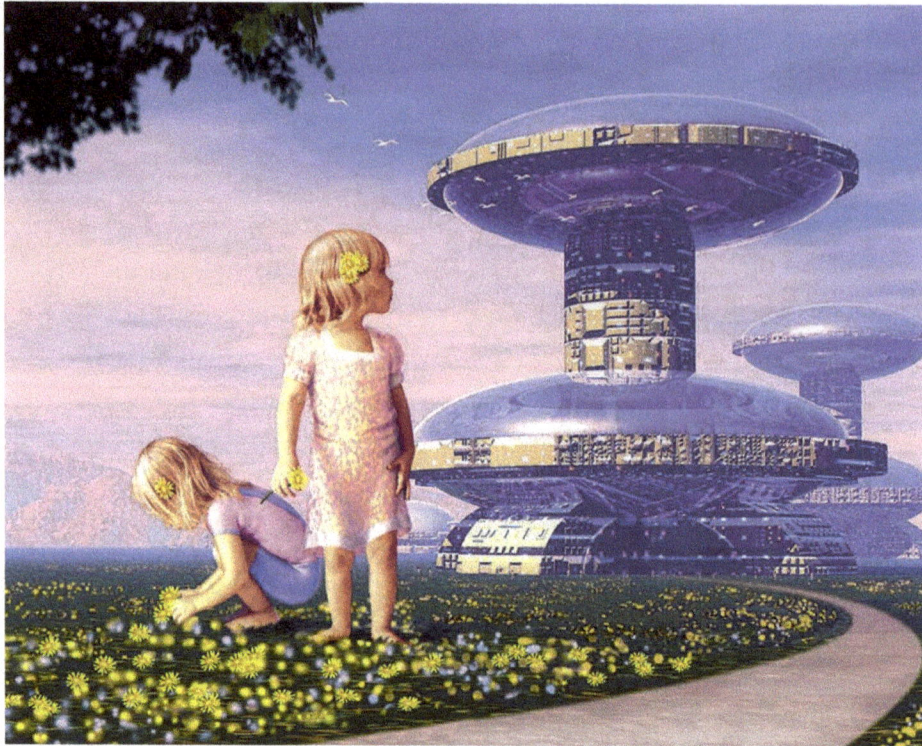

Correspondingly – the rejuvenating by means of the proposed concentration according to clinical scores or just for rejuvenation of the physical body can be applied as many times as you like or need, and every man will determine the age at which he is comfortable to live by himself.

Information on methods of rejuvenation can be complemented from the lecture by Grabovoi G. P. of 20 November 2001:

"And here from the point of view of rejuvenation, in order the rejuvenation exists in the presence of natural development of reality – rejuvenation can be considered as the next evolution of the cellular composition. And then no contradiction here arises.

Here the rejuvenation is just a manifestation of the structure of the Creator actually here in this point from the point of view of eternal development, and including – that your Consciousness corresponds, for example, in this case to this task.

That is, everyone chooses when to rejuvenate: after, for example, there, 70 years, or before, or, there, in some age that is, well, considered constantly like medium young. That is, some system is selected for each person.

And there really exists such an element when others possess as if a capability to age.

It turns out that in terms of the organization of the whole Collective Consciousness, in order to have some earlier point of rejuvenation, here then you need to be able to actually transfer the knowledge to others: either, well, just to rejuvenate foremost those who you meet, according to control, or to teach there, right?..

But in some cases sometimes – for example, according to clinical scores – as if very radical rejuvenating is acceptable, which is fixed at once in outward appearance, for example, by other people, and maybe even to such an extreme, well, level that it is immediately evident that man became younger for many years".

In the Teachings "On salvation and harmonious development" very much attention is given to rejuvenating in various works of Grigori Grabovoi.

Rejuvenating Through the Novelty of Perception and a Photo

The theme of rejuvenating is new every day, because man sooner or later starts to think about his appearance and not only about it: rejuvenating is health, good well-being, joy of life and really the novelty of perception.

We often look at old photos and we like ourselves there. Why? Why do we like ourselves there? First, there was really the norm of health there most often, as well as the norm of events. Secondly, there were people there who were the

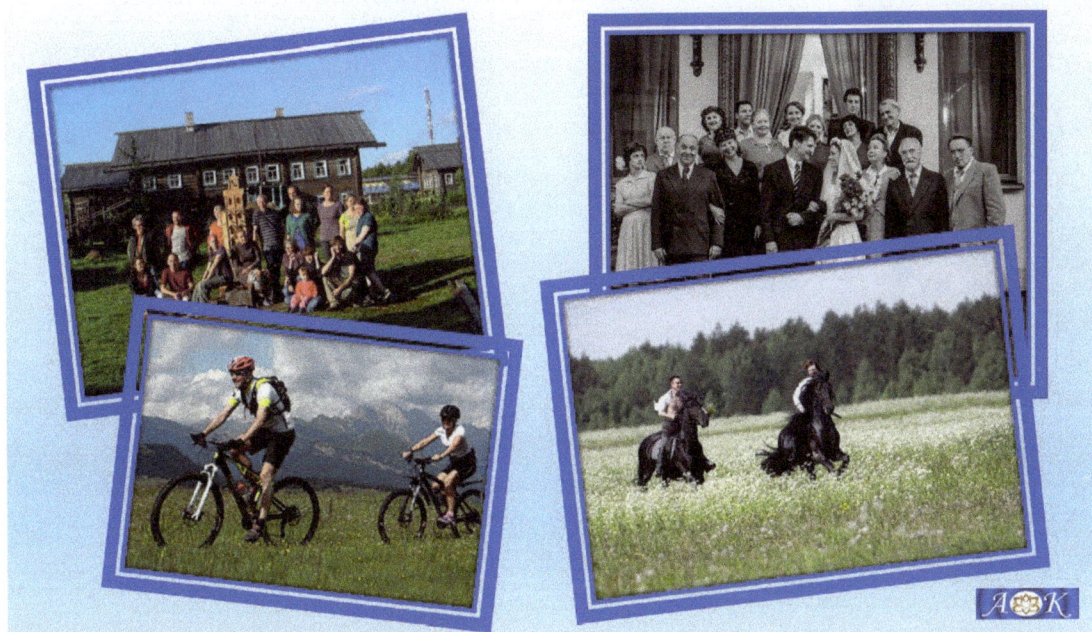

witnesses of our good state there.

Therefore, using the knowledge of Grigori Grabovoi about the novelty of perception, one can reflect on the physical environment where the photo is, can understand – WHAT exactly has been superimposed on this photo, what events of external reality. Only after that it is possible to enter the subsystem of the photo itself for the process of rejuvenating.

The extract from the workshop of Grigori Petrovich Grabovoi "Teachings of Grigori Grabovoi about God. Methods of Eternal Life" of June 4, 2005 as if introduces us into the process of rejuvenating in the technologies of eternal development.

"That is, the following axiom of development in the technologies of eternal development, and at the same time as if growing – this technology - into, namely into the method: the creation of novelty of perception – here you can see the same picture well in the usual way, and it can be perceived as a new picture, right? – that is, through the wave of novelty, although the landscape may be the same, for example the natural landscape.

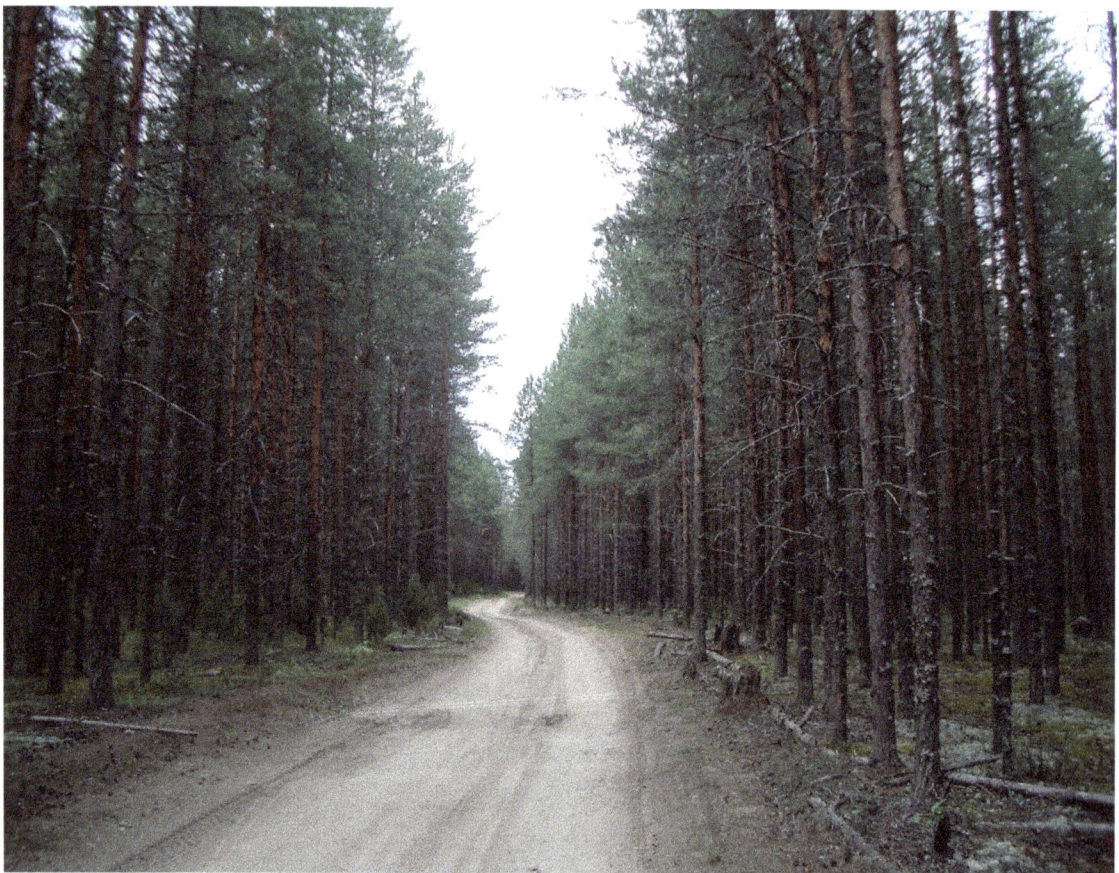

Here you have a familiar street for a long time, you have been walking over it for, for example, ten years, but at some point you can create novelty.

And by the way, at the time of creation of novelty the regeneration of organism structure happens, that is the organism actually returns on the information to the level of an earlier perception. So, in the technologies of eternal life, it is often necessary to actually rejuvenate, right? or as if there – it`s *even possible to call – as if to adjust, perhaps, from the point of view that, like in complex systems: it is the orientation to a stable state – it is the norm.*

How man can know that he develops eternally? He has to understand very clearly that he can enter his original state, when he had the norm there. Many people have norm all the time, for example, right?.. Then, it turns out here, there is just the highlighting of some areas as if on purpose, that is, an elementary action - a person takes a photo or recalls: then there was the norm. And he as if enters this state, takes the wave.

But here the attraction of novelty of perception is a special technology especially in working with the photosystems. Because the photographic image is differ by the fact that as soon as there is a photo, the events of external reality accumulate, as if the outer layer of information. So you need also to go as if to a subsystem, as if to the physical environment itself – which is called photo.

It turns out that when a control does for a photo, then it turns out that the novelty is quite complicated system for such a simple thing as a photo. It is better to work through the thought forms and perception of some plots of there, well, natural environment, of static scenes: the forest, well, a kind of a road, for example, and so on."

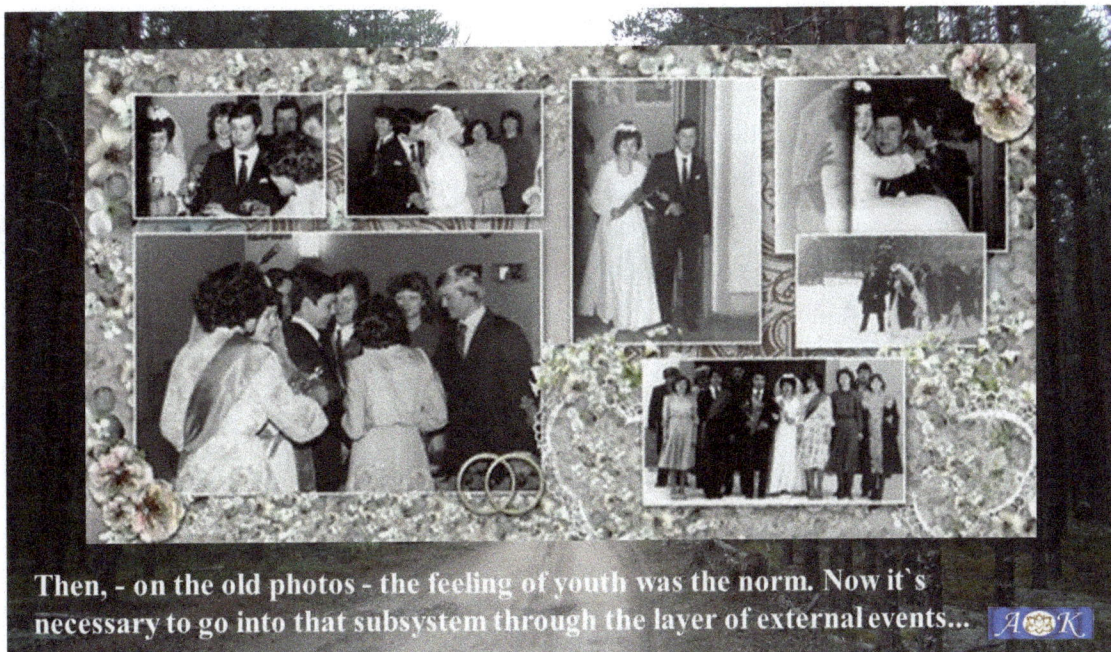

Then, - on the old photos - the feeling of youth was the norm. Now it`s necessary to go into that subsystem through the layer of external events...

Short lecture extract may, of course, give an understanding of the process, but if you perceive all the methods, given in the seminar, the particular method is then easily understood. You just have to perceive the knowledge given by Grigori Grabovoi without effort, because the knowledge is transmitted so that the knowledge is yours, that is of the person who perceives it, and he as if already knows it. Why he knows? Because he was already thinking over his old photos, but didn`t just go there, to the subsystem, and now he can easily come to remember the norm.

The novelty of perception means to perceive that time by other way, to understand the beauty and joy of the events, to find that state of youth, happiness, and health. And the state is quickly found, the cells perceive it, because then it was the norm. You just need to add to the perception of the old photos a bit of knowledge that gives Grigori Grabovoi. And that's all!

January 9, 2017.

Direct Access to the Event Structure to Restore Health. Cure testimonial

5 November, 2016.

On the eve I had a long walk with my grandchildren – we went to the green area, somehow to dispel the autumn greyness. In the forest, there are no chemicals scattered on the sidewalks, but just all around the land there is still like a thin layer of airy snow. The kids were eager to make a snowman but the snow was loose and not sticky. I had to make a something like a snowman with funny ears made of leaves on a bench.

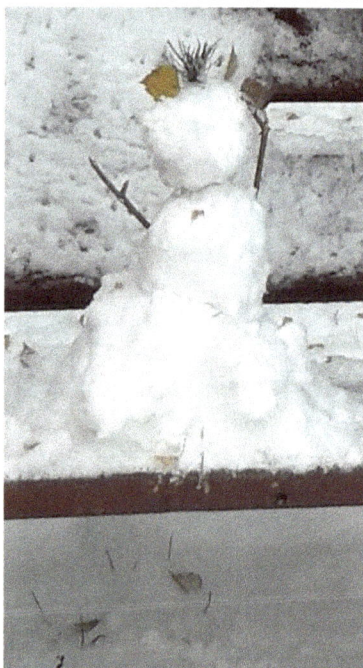

The result of the walks affected directly – the nose responded to festivities, mostly rather to clothes: the back was feeling somehow unpleasantly and chilly... It was on November 4th.

On November 5th the variant of the disease manifested itself more clearly with simply running nose and periodic sneezing. I decided that the script should be turned in the opposite direction of development – in the direction of recovery norm. Once I applied good restoration technology for the throat, then the disease was gone immediately. Here it was necessary to change the areas of numbers allocation, it was necessary to find them exactly, which is the most difficult thing in this technology, because the rest is already attained, and the Spirit remembers the result.

Thus, the number 1 – the number of macro salvation should be placed in the field of the disease and lit with the silvery light. I did everything in my physical body. Since the "flow" was running from some particular area of the nose, then I put the number 1 "one" in the area where there was a reason, supposedly in the sinuses, and gave a bright light.

Next I had to find the way to recovery, restoration, which I specified with the number 2 "two". I placed the "two" nearby my physical body, but very close to the body, so the glow could go immediately onto the cellular structure, i.e. in order the cells could get the norm light. The "two" was light, but not enough to restore health once to the norm. Hence, it is necessary to light the "two"! How?

Highlighting of the "two" – or the path to recovery means highlighting the result. The result in the classical scheme of Grigori Grabovoi's technologies is specified with figure 3.

In this technology "three" is located on the luminous column on the right and front of the body – it's a controlling construction – it is necessary to start moving the number 3 at a given speed up along the infinite column. The column is vertical and infinite. We show our result to the whole world in our perception,

Direct access to the event structure to restore health

1 – the number of macro salvation should be placed in the field of the disease

2 – number sense is full recovery, health

Number "two" with maximum of light is a complete control loop.

3 – it's a controlling construction

© Grabovoi G.P., 2002

we show it on this column as the digit 3. The "three" is moving as the rheostat slider along the luminous column.

Once accepted, the number 2 starts lightening because of the number 3 motion and we get control. Number "two" with maximum of light is a complete control loop. Naturally, that's necessary to know a reverse impulse and control the process on the physical plane. The process of control is based on the light principles. All the outer systems are affected due to the glow, in this case there is such a principle, as when a person is healthy.

In the given control, the location of the number "three" could be heard, that is, the exact location was designated as if there was a sparkling touch, or a sound, like burning Bengal fire, could be heard. The exact location of the number "three" was found, and that led to the bright light of the number "two" in front of the physical body. There is a cure process – for a while it is necessary to hold the illuminated figure "two". Control is complete.

Everything was going during the lunch time period. At about 5 p.m. there were no longer any effects of cold, there was no sneezing, nose breathing was smooth and calm. Thanks to Grigori Grabovoi for plain and simple rescue salvation technologies.

This technology is described by the Author in a seminar: "Grabovoi G.P., Methods of control by means of own Consciousness, based on the structure of perception to regulate the system for prevention of macro catastrophe and direct access to the event structure", May 23, 2002.

Remove Negative Information from Events

The situations with some coughing, tingling may be often repeated, and sometimes a human may get it. It is necessary to develop a method for yourself to normalize these events, so the situation would not linger on in space and time.

For example, some event indicates that you should pay attention to it. You may not unpack, unzip the event, but practice with just information. What shall we be doing? The event itself is naturally neither deleted nor disbanded, but just elicit the negative component out of it, and send it into the area where this information transformation occurs. A portal, which is located in a small sphere at a distance of 1.8 m from your right shoulder forward has this kind of characteristic.

CONSTANT OUTPUT OF NEGATIVE INFORMATION AFTER ANY OPERATION

All work is performed only in the positive direction for yourself and for all through the macro salvation level. To do as the Creator makes, and He always makes universally and for all.

1,8 meters

The output is better made through the so called "portal", which is a point located opposite the right shoulder at a distance of 1.8m. The negative is removed there in the point. Transformation occurs there in the point, and that is the feature of this point.

19751 – negative output after any operation: number series is located in the portal (a point, sphere), then you begin stretching the information threads of the negative out of you with the help of the number series up to discoloration. Transformation takes place right in the portal.

On the Teaching materials of Grigori Grabovoi

19751 – an output of negative after any work: a number series is placed in the portal (e.g. a point, a small sphere), and then you start using the number series to pull out the information negative threads from yourself up to their discoloration. Transformation occurs exactly in the portal, that is its property.

For example, on September 1st, 2016 some tingling was felt in the muscle of the right leg, as well as there was some point pain in the knee. It was happening during the trip, that is why the Portal method was applied right when moving in the tube/metro. When a small sphere is taken, and it is assigned to be the portal in the exact coordinate, then it is always clear that this technology according to the Teaching of Grigori Grabovoi is exactly what is required to rescue everyone including myself.

Then the number series 741 was applied, which has the following characteristic: the norm of all events (hence, including the norm of my events too). Only the negative area was allocated from the information in the tingling space, and it had to be pulled out with that number series into a small sphere. That time it seemed to be like a small gray ball with needles (but not sharp), it seemed to be rolling along the beam from the number series into the small portal sphere opposite the right shoulder. It was enough to bring a ball to the portal, then the actions occurred themselves. It has already been practiced, it is not necessary to think over it.

The number series "worked" hard, the beam was adjusted not immediately, but anyhow, information was being deleted. Then I used another number series: 19751 – a number series of an instant action. Using those two series I pulled the

The technology can be used to practice with the following number series:

39751831 - intoxication;

1,8 meters

91981371 – an output of negative information;

7794218 – remove social virus through a joint level;
7794218 – elimination of viruses

On the Teaching materials of Grigori Grabovoi

negative out of those events, which as if were transmitting the signals. In the evening, and even more so the next day tingling in my legs was gone.

The same technology can be used to practice with the following number series:

7794218 – remove social virus through a joint level;

7794218 – elimination of viruses;

91981371 – an output of negative information;

39751831 – intoxication;

Note that events are not disbanded, and only a negative part of the event is taken out from information.

Work with an Aggressive Person Using the Number Series 14789

According to the lectures of G. P. Grabovoi "Teaching about God. System of the prevention of terrorism" of 15.09.2004

Number series on the contour of a person creates the norm of peace – it is the norm of his life, the norm of events development. Then the events of his past turn off into the norm of the following actions: he starts to look for the ways out

Work with an aggressive person using the number series 14789
According to the lecture of G.P.Grabovoi "Teaching about God. The system of the prevention of terrorism" of 09.15.2004

1 - at the level of the right shoulder

Number series on the contour of a person creates the norm of peace – it is the norm of his life, the norm of events development. Then the events of his past turn off into the norm of the following actions: he starts to look for the ways out of the situation.

The numbers 14789 rigidly fix the level of the norm.

The figure of the representative of the aggressive party

Phase of the exact stability in collective control

9 – at the level of the left heel

© Grabovoi G.P., 2004

of the situation.

Restoring the Source System to Receive Information

Question: *"In some domestic action there is a repetition of the same information that was in the past. How to remove it?"*

G.P. Grabovoi`s answer:

"If you have the repetition of the same information in action, you need to move to the internal structure of the Soul, that is, in the part where the Soul connects with the physical body, and examine – is it consciously, that is, if your personality keeps this information in special way from the point of view of the need to react to it?

Or is it the information, which is not of such a fundamental level, but simply delayed in the structure of exchange processes of information – as if unnecessary, interfering structure?

In the second case – if this is unnecessary structure – you can just use the number series 49181. It allows normalizing, that is restoring the source system to receive information.

This number series is possible, by the way, to be used in the cases when you develop a filter, which assumes the information from eternity. That is, the number allows normalizing any level of the receiver of information".

Grigori Grabovoi: "The Teachings of Grigori Grabovoi about God. Technology of memory development to ensure eternal life", November 9, 2015.

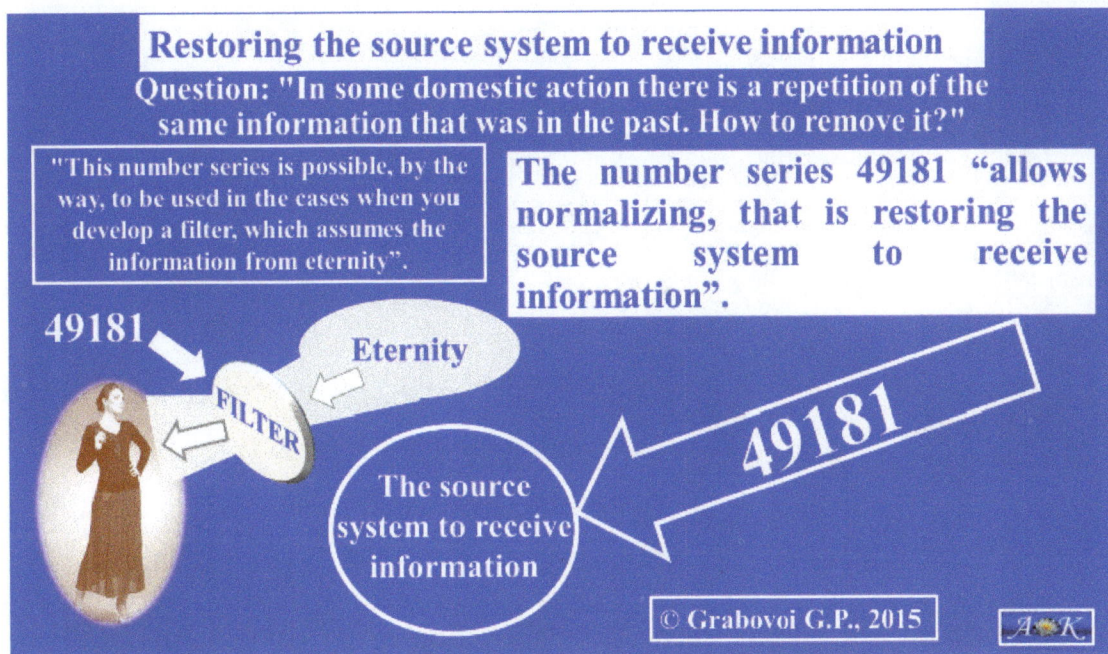

Restoring the source system to receive information

Question: "In some domestic action there is a repetition of the same information that was in the past. How to remove it?"

"This number series is possible, by the way, to be used in the cases when you develop a filter, which assumes the information from eternity".

The number series 49181 "allows normalizing, that is restoring the source system to receive information".

49181

Eternity

FILTER

The source system to receive information

49181

© Grabovoi G.P., 2015

Recovery Impulse from Palms of Child

The 30th of August 2016 I heard my child coughing. Put him next to me and explained that it is necessary to be able to restore one`s health. How is it possible to do?

For example: you can mentally send an impulse from your left palm into your right palm. This impulse contains salvation of everybody including yourself, so – it contains the norm of health at once.

Now we have to send the impulse from the right palm into the area of implementation (Our Consciousness is constructed in such a way that what we declare, there we go). We find the area of implementation in the infinitely remote region; we find it with our Consciousness.

Child is told that the impulse is such little light vertical column, so it moves in space, finding the desired area of implementation, where the child is healthy.

The path of the impulse can be tracked and this movement can be seen. As soon as you got into this area, there is a reverse impulse from out of it, the light goes to that point of the body, which is problematic at the moment, which requires attention, recovery.

Grandson actually saw the back bright column of light that came to him, and was very happy.

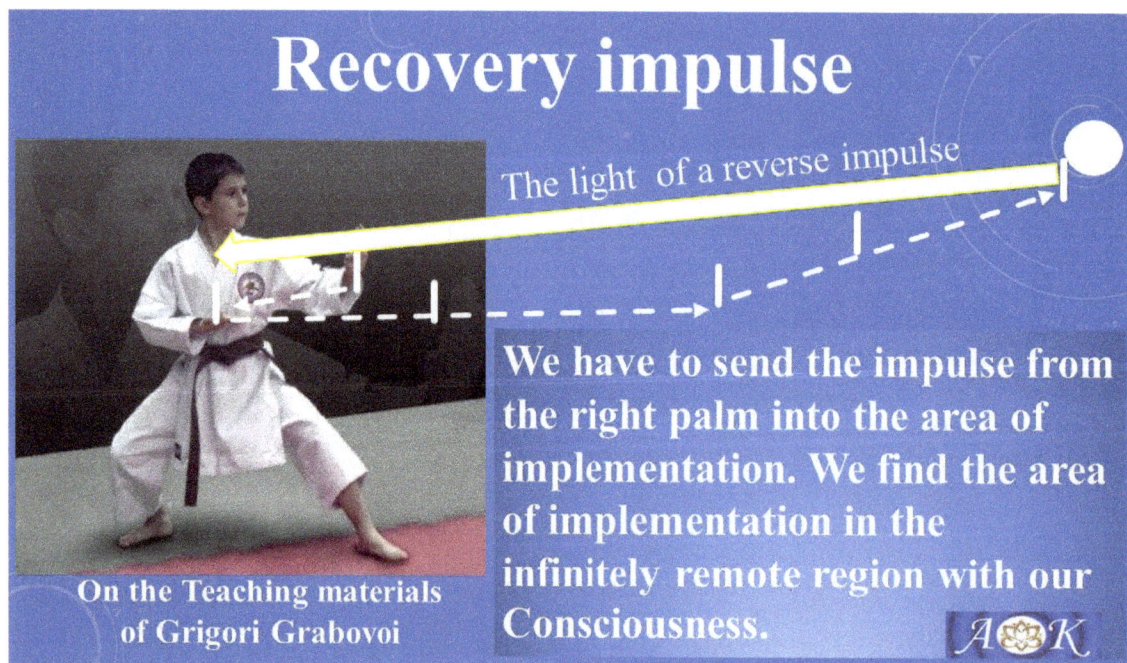

Recovery impulse

The light of a reverse impulse

We have to send the impulse from the right palm into the area of implementation. We find the area of implementation in the infinitely remote region with our Consciousness.

On the Teaching materials of Grigori Grabovoi

Why do we use palms? Why does the impulse go from palms? Because then it is clear that this is that physical body that needs help. So, if a person is working on the restoration of his health, he needs to look at his palms. That's all.

The joint level – control was implemented from his palms: the child did and Control specialist did out of child`s palms. Together they traced the path of the impulse to the area of implementation. And the receipt of back impulse was voiced by the child.

This technology is from the workshop of Grigori Petrovich Grabovoi "Teaching of Grigori Grabovoi about God. Control by controlling impulse", of April 11, 2005.

"But it is better periodically to bring control up to complete control – where did the specific beam of Light disappear, which came from you? where is it? what is its source? what are its links? which contacts? – and so on. When you start to monitor this area at the level of action, then in principle you always understand what happens on with the process, if you treat somebody, yes?.. for example, there treatment".

"And here you can see that your action in the primary impulse is a clear/transparent value. That is when you personally do the action, you are working in a transparent system of coordinates".

How the World Speaks with Us. Testimonial

On September 19th, 2016 I went to the doctor to get consulting. It was assumed that it would be the last consultation examination, because it was time to go back to norm. As always, I carried out both general and local control while moving. One of the repetitive control is macro salvation in every point of space-time with the personal objective in the center of this point.

This is a common scheme, and the specific one will be shown below. The fact is that the goal is not to show exactly the technology, but the goal is to show getting into the mutual control, technology is a method: to make as the Creator does.

If to consider the control scheme, then it is very clear:

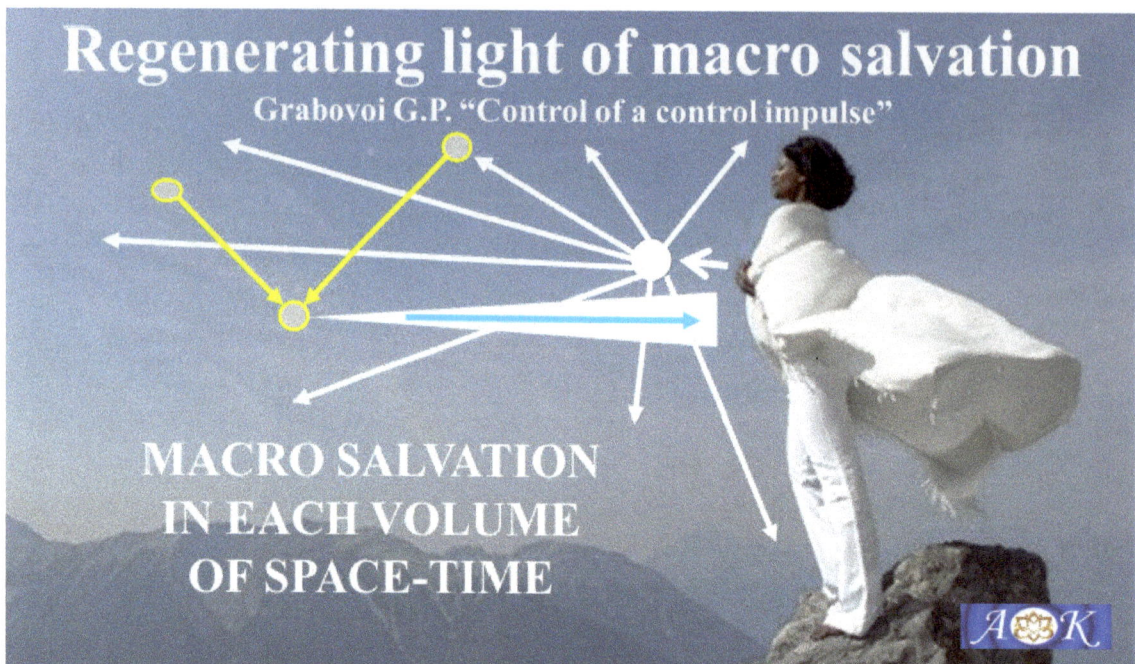

Regenerating light of macro salvation
Grabovoi G.P. "Control of a control impulse"

MACRO SALVATION
IN EACH VOLUME
OF SPACE-TIME

First, I made a slight control on the transfer of the Teaching Knowledge. Somehow, my attention was attracted by a young man who walked into the subway car and put his suitcase so that the suitcase was constantly falling. It had just to be turned with the other side, then the suitcase would not have fallen, but the young man preferred to keep it himself. I transferred him knowledge mentally in his hands, while getting the knowledge into the sphere of the Teaching Knowledge. Then he sat down on the outer seat and pressed his suitcase with the elbow. His hands were already free, only the elbow was occupied. One more characteristic feature – he was with his wife, but did not call her to sit nearby, although the close seat was vacant. They left at the same station as I ...

So, after the transfer of knowledge, I began observing the level of macro salvation with the norm of my health at the center of each point, that is, I had to find the reverse impulse by combining luminous points. And what was amazing? That point, which a reverse impulse beam went from was shining very brightly, it was not necessary to look for it, that was so bright that the beam from it directed at any part of my body or the whole body. Control was carried out easily and accurately.

I describe the event that happened yesterday, but and today I also see clearly the point from which there is a return impulse. This is an amazing state, it is possible to re-enter it again, because the spiritual state has stored.

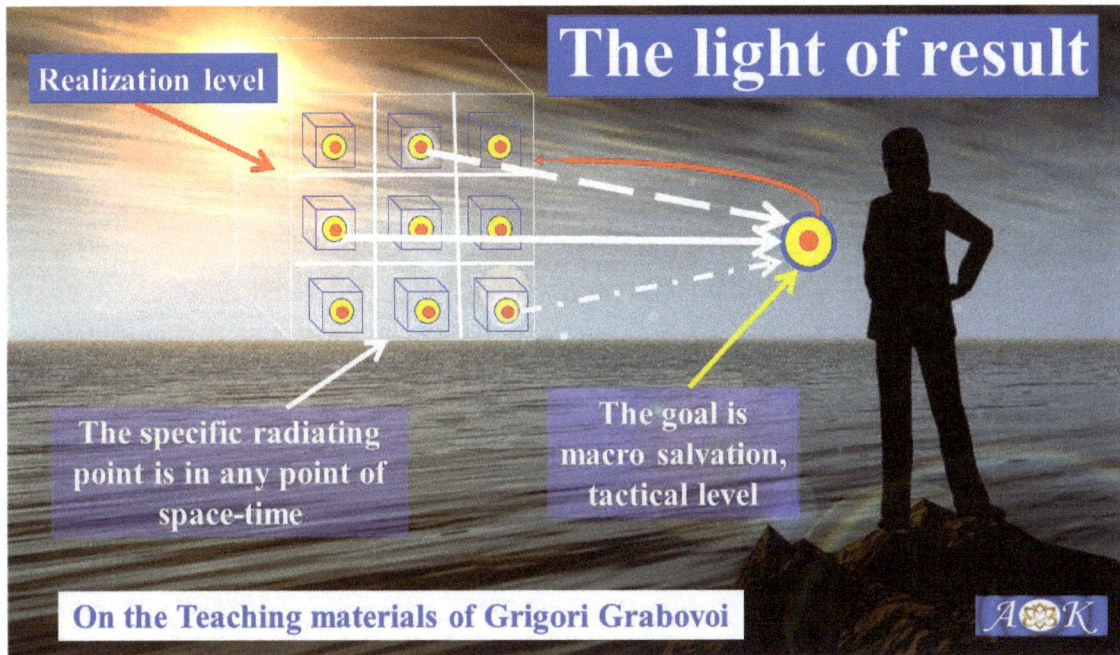

The light of result

Realization level

The specific radiating point is in any point of space-time

The goal is macro salvation, tactical level

On the Teaching materials of Grigori Grabovoi

Grigori Grabovoi states during his seminar dated June 8th, 2001: *"You, in principle, firstly restore it <the impulse>, then perceive it. Why restore? Because the Creator has created it in the future"*.

It turns out that by passing Knowledge to that man, at once I restored the impulse for myself. It means that the Knowledge transfer activates accuracy in controlling in the level of macro salvation. In practice, it turned that way.

Outcome: consultation was held on a very high level, by hand I was got into different consulting rooms, and the examination showed that the norm rate for a

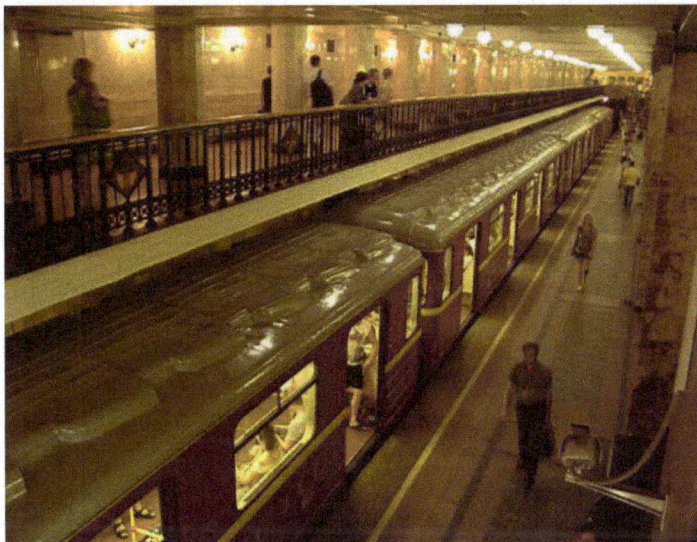

particular event at that stage was reached. I received recommendations and said goodbye with gratitude to the clinic personnel.

In addition, I introduce a part of the control scheme according to Grabovoi G.P.'s technology from the lecture dated April 11th, 2005.

In the event there was one more interesting sign: when we got into the subway car (in front of me there was a couple with the falling suitcase), then next station was announced as if from the other end of the subway line, as if the train moved in the opposite direction. It was a surprise, and then we all smiled. It turned out that the reality showed immediately a possible option of the scheme – a very precise one, by the way: to restore the reverse impulse, which had already been created by the Creator (as we have begun to move forward to the end station, but the subway station was named already as if from a place of the train's arrival).

At the next station the driver corrected the announcement, and then everything was as usual. You probably just have to see the world more accurately, to "hear" all the tips and not to miss in space a clearly falling suitcase, because it is in our perception, we were "given" to understand.

The Technology of the Gold Ball. You Need to Find a Way

Grigori Grabovoi in the seminar "Teaching of Grigori Grabovoi about God. Dynamic structuring of the Soul" gave a fabulous technology. "Fabulous technology" – means that it is in the Russian folk tales, but in the seminar the exact controlling method is given. The method is following:

"That is why, for example, you can go through the ball of these relationships – that's how linear systems are wrapped into the sphere and you always find a way, for example there in space, right? If you are in the city, in a country place where you need to find a way, it`s very simple – take the exit to Golden spectrum. And where on a silver background Golden spectrum according to the target tasks occur, then, in principle, it is a place, as a rule, or a place of control, or a specific place, well, which you need, right?.. physically that is". © Grabovoi G.P., 2004

The technology of the gold ball from the seminar of November 24, 2004 is easily perceived if to adapt it to the specific conditions. First, it is easy to recall, and secondly, to understand and the most important – the result can be received very fast.

27 August 2016 a young woman went to the forest to pick mushrooms. It was in the afternoon (after a late lunch), so she said she would go alone and not for long. It took some time. The children began to worry and miss their mom, although they had their own affairs and fun. It had to call and know how she was and where she was and to tell that she had to actually go back.

It turned out that she lost the way back, came back twice in a familiar place, but couldn`t find the swamp she needed through which there was a path. In

Russia it's called "leads down" and more often it happens in the swamp. It was necessary to urgently take some actions. Screaming – the forest deafens the sound, although she had heard a dog barking. There was nothing but just to switch on a car horn: it is heard in the forest, but all the neighbors can hear that a car buzzes for some reason. So it was decided not to switch on the signal.

The phone was put down, and then a place in the middle of the garden plot for control was found. The 8-years old child helped to do control. He was just doing what his grandma told. And they did the following: they immediately found the young woman in the forest on information level and showed her on a silver background the golden spot where she had to go. They pronounced that she knew where to step, which way to go, and in generally she had to know the way home.

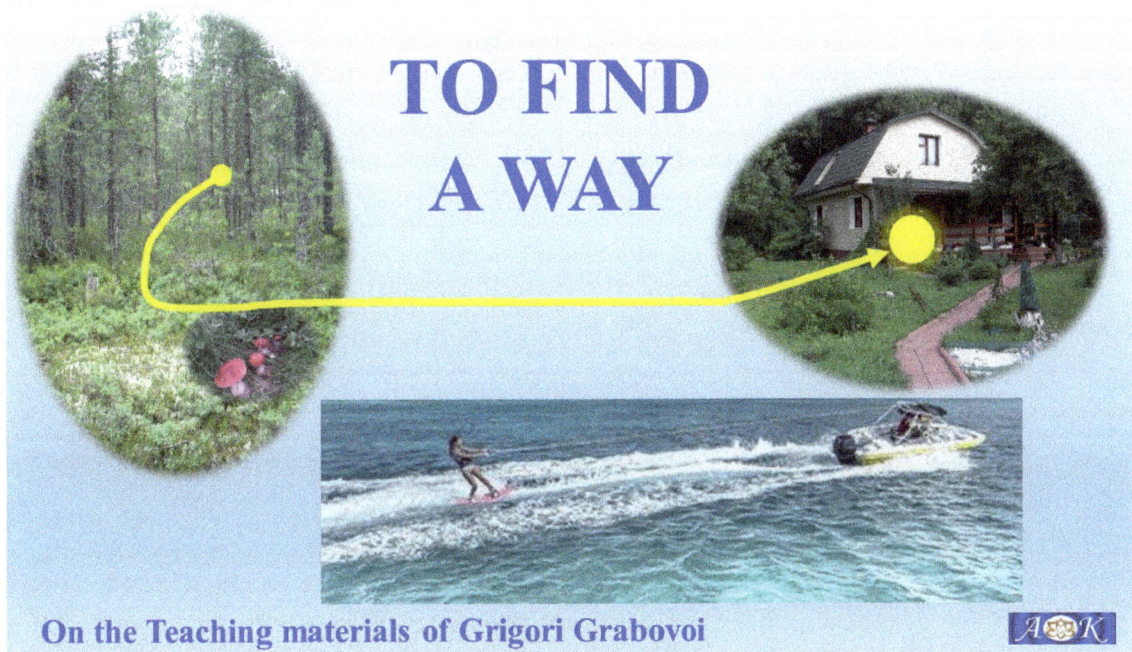

On the Teaching materials of Grigori Grabovoi

Further, there was made the adaptation to the current situation: a golden thread was given in the hands of the young woman, and the ball was in the center of the garden plot. She was pulled out of the woods with this thread. It turns out that the light of the ball was in the country house. The grandson then told his grandmother that it was like the fact that from the boat on the lake a rope was thrown to a water skier and a boat pulled a skier behind him. Grandmother and grandchild were as if on the boat. One can say like this. What is most important – he helped his mom to get out of the forest.

When it became clear that the control was done, they took the phone and called.

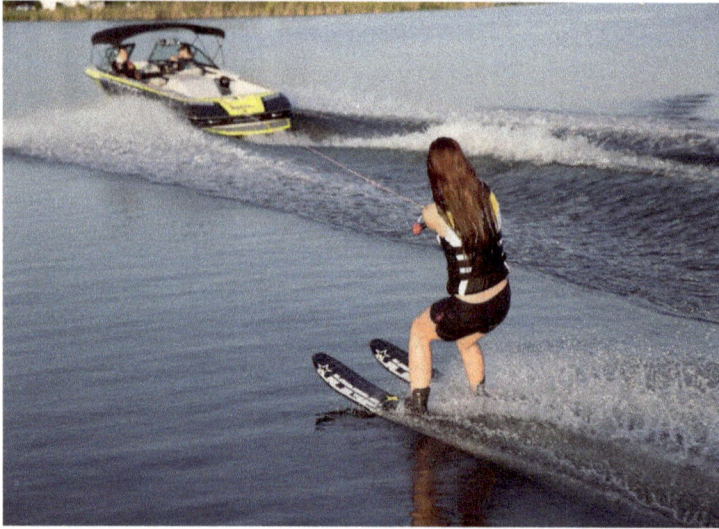

It was now possible to determine from which side was the sun, where was the swamp, how many fallen trees were and so on – the purpose was just to talk. The sound of the voice continued to pull, like a golden thread.

By the way, the place for control, as we see from the mentioned technology, also had to be found, and it was found immediately. They were contacting by phone until the young woman came to the fence of garden plots. It took already little time. She came out not by the usual way, but through fallen trees, through impassable thickets, but there were no scratches on her. She brought a full basket of mushrooms, including a lot of ceps. The children were happy to see their mom, because the sunset was already dangerously close...

Level of control? This is the level of macrosalvation, the level of assistance to everyone, the level of eternity – the man must live and grow and not be lost in the woods. Everyone defines his own wording, finds the explanation for his actions, seeking additional resources in the control.

Thanks to Grigori Grabovoi because HE gives SUCH KNOWLEDGE that helps to develop own creativity including.

How to Help Those People Who Have Lost
From the experience of application of the

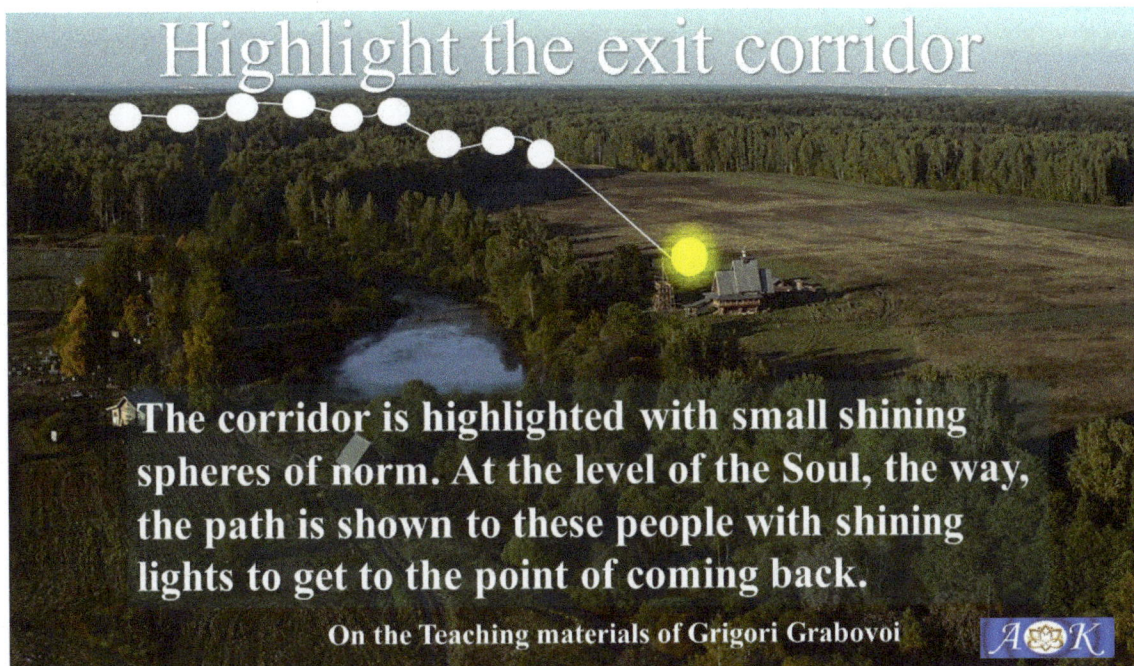

Highlight the exit corridor

The corridor is highlighted with small shining spheres of norm. At the level of the Soul, the way, the path is shown to these people with shining lights to get to the point of coming back.

On the Teaching materials of Grigori Grabovoi

authorized technologies of Grigori Grabovoi.

Technologies were formulated and issued by Antonina Kravtsova on September 09th, 2016.

Option 1.

Find people, who have lost, at the information level.

Allocate and highlight these people in your Consciousness. With this action we help ALL, who were lost (Macro level), including these lost people. Highlight the exact coordinate, place, point where they should get out to, come back. This point should be highlighted strongly, and we practice from it.

Highlight the exit corridor. Visualize how people are moving along this corridor in light. The corridor is highlighted with small shining spheres of norm, and every sphere organizes the following norm of event in every three meters in front of those people, who are moving. At the level of the Soul, the way, the path is shown to these people with shining lights to get to the point of coming back. You should visualize how those lost people came back, model the norm, you would be able to see those people in the arrival point, and there should be also something else nearby, for example, the tree.

Option 2.

Use your consciousness to define the leader in the group of lost people. This leader is moving forward and "is able to hear" you. Highlight three sevens – 777 opposite his eyes in blue color, these numbers are a part of the number sequence 31877719113, which is used by the person who carries out control. This number series transfers the right decision, i.e. shows the exit. This technology is universal and can be applied in any other situations. The technology of the "Norm of Flight" created by Grigori Grabovoi on October 09th, 2001 was used in this particular case.

Option 3.

"Getting into the ten".

"Getting into the ten"

Hit 10 in the center of the target to get immediate visualization. The trajectory of an arrow flight is the way and exit for those who are lost.

On the Teaching materials of Grigori Grabovoi

It looks like an arrow flying in the target. Hit 10 in the center of the target to get immediate visualization. The trajectory of an arrow flight is the way and exit

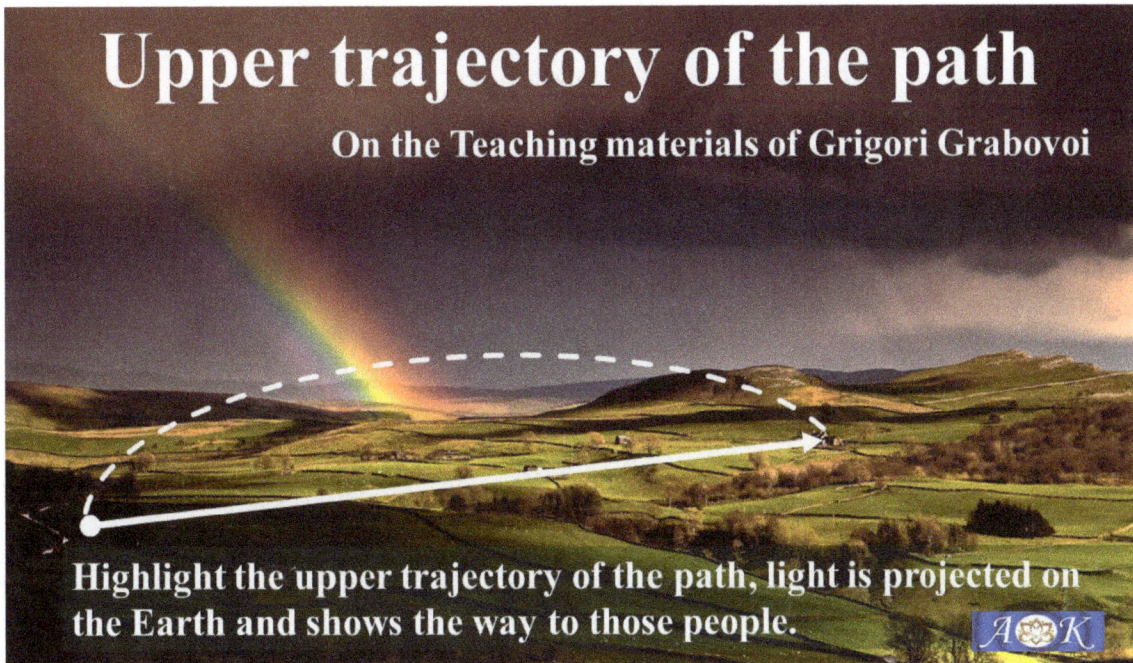

Upper trajectory of the path

On the Teaching materials of Grigori Grabovoi

Highlight the upper trajectory of the path, light is projected on the Earth and shows the way to those people.

for those who are lost. The one who carries out control should visualize the target and the arrow flight, and all the time see these coming back, emerging people and this «10 mark».

Option 4.

You can practice visualization through the huge, vast space of sky above those, who were lost and coming back simultaneously including those who carry out control. Highlight the upper trajectory of the path, light is projected on the Earth and shows the way to those people.

You CAN visualize to help, to pull out people. Carry out control.

The "Eights" Nearby the Sofa
or Exit from Control

Every control process generally has three stages, or it can be split into three controlling stages. The first stage in the input in the level, where man works. To say more precisely, it is access into control structure. Usually access is reached through the allocation of the macro salvation level, but there are also methods, which the one who learns the Teachings of Grigori Grabovoi has learnt from the Teaching materials. For example, there is a special learning course on the materials of Grigori Grabovoi, where it is told about the creation of the spheres of macro salvation, which was given in Russian.

The second stage is the control process on the task, which is implemented, solved at the moment with the help of some technology. At this stage man can see both the controlling process and final result. Here different controlling structures, given in the Teaching, can be used. It is given simply and shown in the materials from the Education Program on the Teaching of Grigori Grabovoi.

The third stage is the result. You may concentrate on it or to see it at once, to prolong the control action and so on. Like in any prayer, there should be the output with the POINT.

So, my sharing and testimony about the third stage.

My friend was staying with me for several days. We had talks and also carried out controls with the technologies of Grigori Petrovich Grabovoi. One evening we had practice on the technology, where the controlling construction was in the form of the number 8 (eight). My attention was distracted by children, that is why the third stage, which we had usually finished together, even when we had different goals and objectives, my friend did not finish.

She went to bed and saw that two "eights" were standing nearby the sofa in full height. Two digits – because there were two goals: the first one was to normalize the cellular structure of her body, and the second one to help her son in one case. She was surprised, closed her eyes and tried to fall asleep. But the dream did not come to her because the "eights" were standing next to the sofa. Usually in controlling she followed my voice, and here she had to recollect what she had to do, so the "eights" would leave her. It was funny and surprising. She could see the control she had carried out before. On the other side, what did the controlling construction want from her?

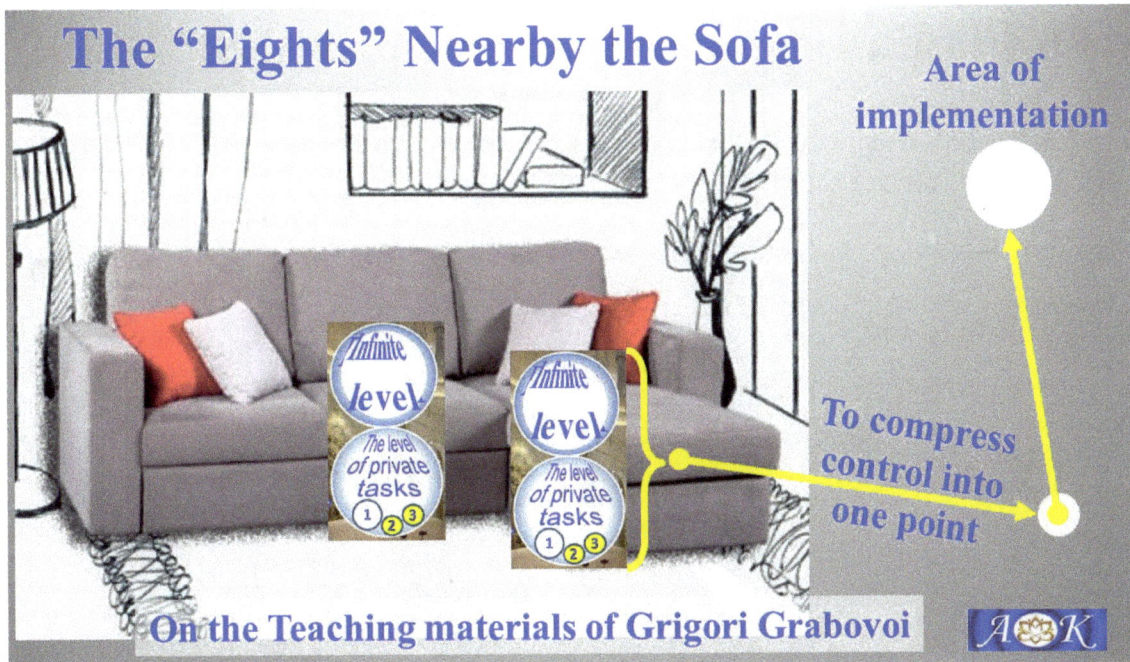

The "Eights" Nearby the Sofa

Area of implementation

Infinite level
The level of private tasks
1 2 3

Infinite level
The level of private tasks
1 2 3

To compress control into one point

On the Teaching materials of Grigori Grabovoi

Later when she told me about it I explained her that she had got the knowledge on control, and she just had to recollect the controlling stages.

And she's got it! What thing? What was the final stage? It is needed to compress the control into one point (compression is also control), and then to send a brightly shining point in the area of implementation, in the infinite remote area, which is seen by the controller usually at once. The back impulse in the form of light comes back to the physical body from the area of implementation. My friend accomplished those actions, the "eights" disappeared from her perception and, she fell asleep.

That is the way how my friend got assistance in the processes of control understanding. It was followed by a good result after her control on the child's health normalization, which was obtained during the doctor's examination of her child. The doctor fixed the norm after child's examination. For sure the result spreads the wings, you get confidence in your actions. And help comes!

Many Thanks to Grigori Grabovoi, HE continues teaching us how to live our life joyfully, with easy-going controlling of events!

November 23, 2016.

To Find a Lost Thing Is a Manifested Result

The knowledge about controllability of the world in the Educational Program on Grigori Grabovoi`s Teachings.

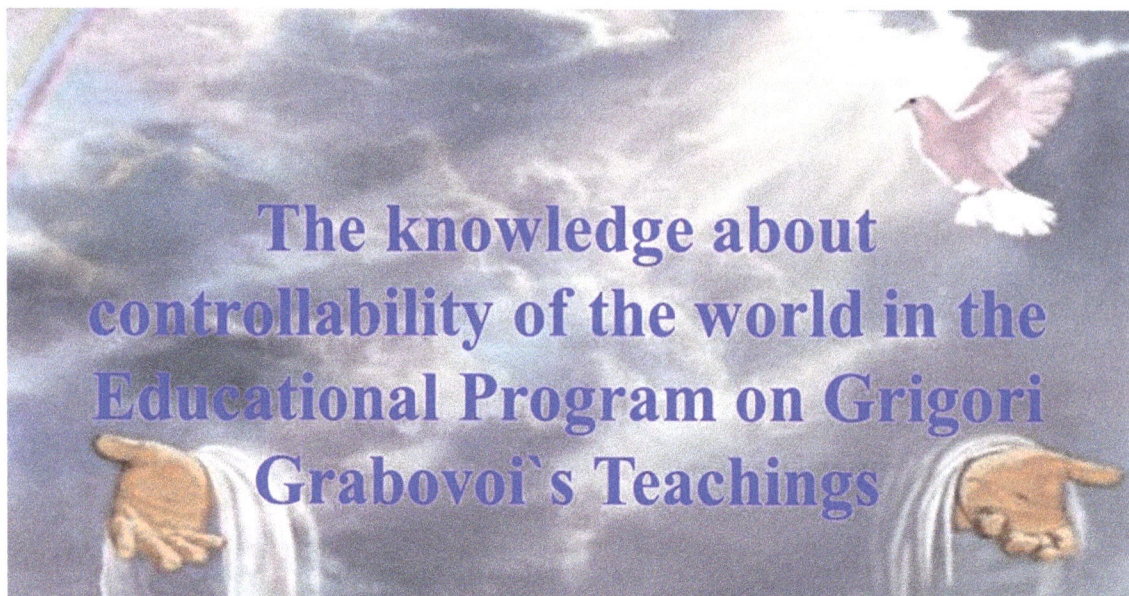

The document "The beginning of the educational program on Grigori Grabovoi`s Teachings" is placed on the website www.grigori-grabovoi.world with the following technology: "Concentration on a point in space improves events or helps you find a lost item after concentration" (https://goo.gl/2i9CzQ).

It turns out that knowledge of carrying out control, of multidimensionality of the world and the issues of crossing of the future with the past may come first, before learning the testimonials and protocols. In spite of the fact that certificates and protocols of works have already been left behind, but I like the proposed concentration, that is why I practiced it periodically. Concentration was made in that way or another one, for example, when information of large space is compressed into the point (a small sphere), but control already goes from this point.

In the article "Dove from Heaven or the Gift of the Kiev Pechersk Saints" the photography plays an important role to describe the object. So, the article was written on May 30th, 2013. And a photo was not available. I had to look through all the albums and view packs of photos. The photo was nowhere to be found. There was a faint hope that I had already scanned it, and it was in the computer database, but ... expectations failed. And then a pause came – a calm state, as if the space was being scanned. And then a clear picture with a photo of a dove emerged in Consciousness. In practice, that was the first time for me: to see clearly and exactly what I was looking for, and to see where it was located. It only remained to take the desired folder with a lecture and get a photo from the file.

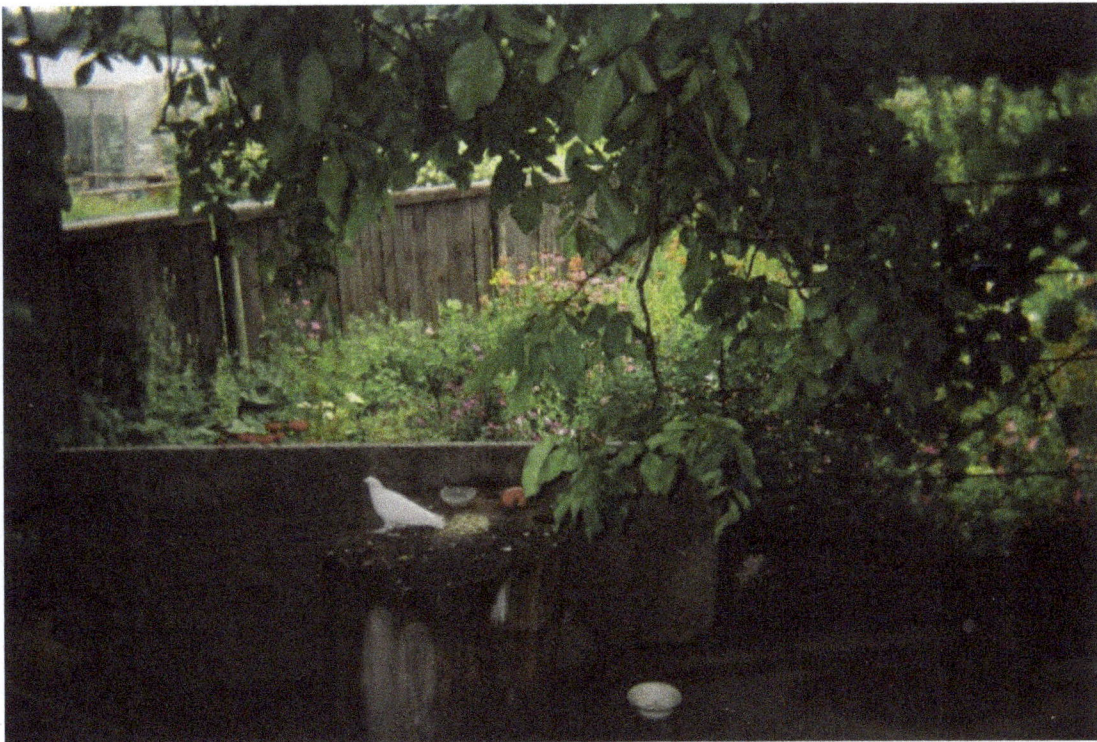

Then everything worked out very well, because the article was published – a pigeon "flew" in the Internet space.

The theory can also be applied, for example, from the seminar on "The Teaching of Grigori Grabovoi about God. Action of Eternal Reality" dated September 8, 2004, which states:

"To get the result for you – this means actually the development of your Soul precisely in the area of spiritual self-awareness. So, you are aware of yourself not just with the Spirit. For the Spirit you are already understandable, in

general, in the first place, namely, there is awareness in terms of the external construction reaction to you: that is, as information of the external world, right?.. generally perceives you in the world as a whole?"

Information of the external World perceived the article on pigeon quite harmoniously, if the dove picture was found. It is a fixed result - the result of the technology application and beginning of the clairvoyance opening particularly according to the Teaching of Grigori Grabovoi.

Snowball

On October 13, 2015 Grigori Grabovoi showed the technology: how to implement and ensure eternal life by means of change in form. The change of form implies a controlling structure, such as a sphere, including a form of thought as well.

"Snowball" is a very good name for this technology, as the work is really carried out with the form of a snowball.

This technology can be adapted, for example, to the specific forecast for the next year – you just need to remember that the next year is some part of eternal life, that the events have already got a start and will be in progress after our control.

You can imagine that in a chain of events of our life there is a ball of snow, where there are all the events of external reality, and the events refer to the specific year – 2017.

Then diagnose this imagined snowball on the subject of the existence of "own personal events in all the phenomena of infinite reality, and it is necessary to take into account that we are talking about infinite events of your personal life" – according to the Author of this technology.

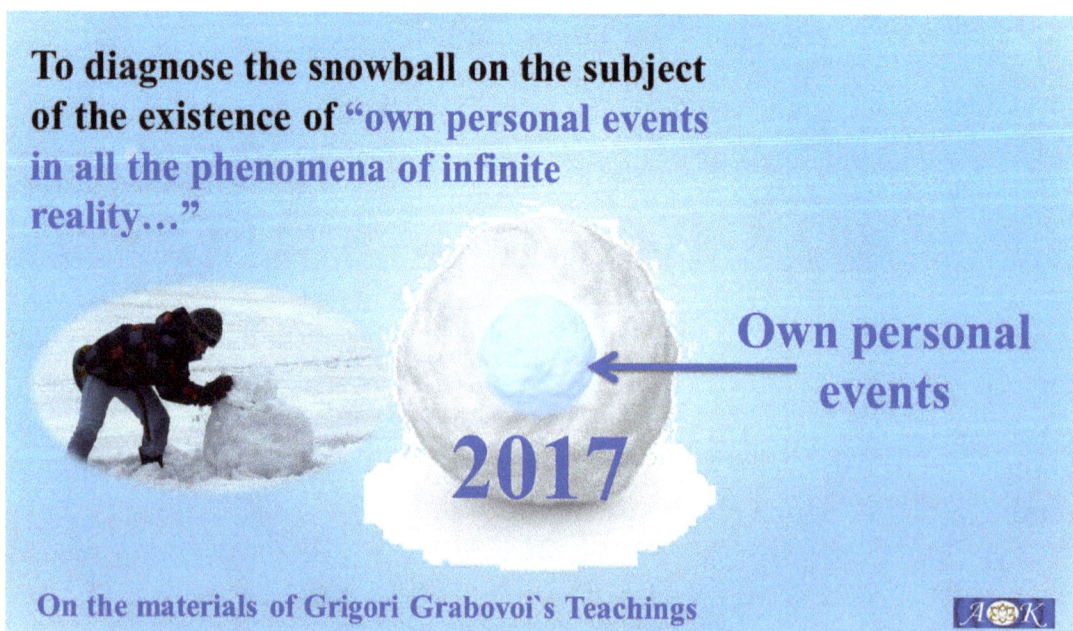

To diagnose the snowball on the subject of the existence of "own personal events in all the phenomena of infinite reality…"

Own personal events

2017

On the materials of Grigori Grabovoi`s Teachings

Everyone can imagine some specific events in reality because life goes on, events unfold in time and space including this specific year 2017.

Then imagine that we come up to and withdraw the amount of snow that refers to our events from this snowball. Then we put this amount of snow in the form of a small ball on the big ball.

This change in shape is the shape of two spheres.

If to imagine that there is no snow inside of a large ball, it is hollow inside, then the part of snow which contains our events, which is in the form of a small snow ball, corresponding to our infinite life events in specific 2017, can be placed inside the ball. Then a small white sphere will shine on the entire inner surface of the large ball.

It turns out that this little sphere is connected with all the world events.

The motion of this sphere inside a large ball can change the events of the outer world and at the same time changes the event structure of human thinking as the person does these actions by means of thinking. And we need to imagine that the entire inner surface of the ball is the events of the whole external reality.

Grigori Petrovich says: "The man upped and passed this sphere with the events of his personal life or with the events of the personal life of another person in respect of whom he carries out control to ensure eternal life inside this large ball with his hand."

You can even visualize that man just took and compacted snow with his hand, having pressed this snow against the inner surface of the ball.

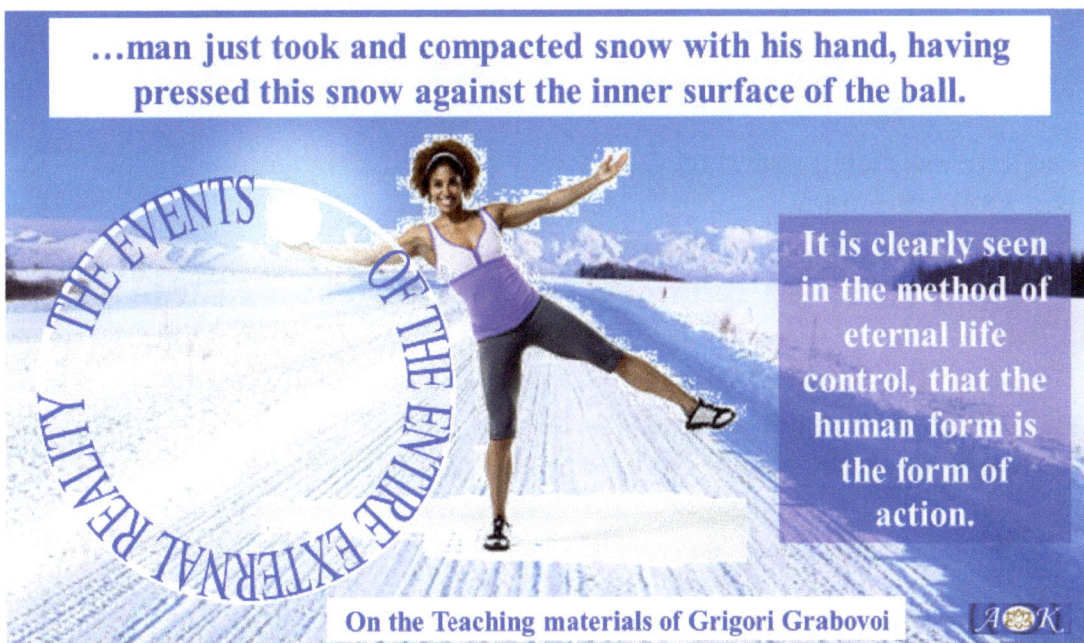

...man just took and compacted snow with his hand, having pressed this snow against the inner surface of the ball.

THE EVENTS OF THE ENTIRE EXTERNAL REALITY

It is clearly seen in the method of eternal life control, that the human form is the form of action.

On the Teaching materials of Grigori Grabovoi

It is clearly seen in the method of eternal life control, that the human form is the form of action.

Having combined one's personal experiences with all the phenomena of infinite reality, the person can complete his actions for the control of eternal life in this way... Description of the Author's technology from the webinar of Grigori Grabovoi, dated October 13, 2015.

It's possible to go further in this control and to consider the events of external reality on the internal surface of the ball, which are advisable to pay attention to next year. There are a lot of options here. You can, for example, visualize that a white shining ball of your events easily rolled around all the events of the next year, so it moves around the inner surface of a big ball and additionally highlights necessary events of the external reality, the important events connected with your personal life. You are even able to see some events, and that will be the connection with reality.

As we have already imagined that a small white sphere shines overall the inner surface of the big ball, then you may not roll the sphere it around the surface, but just visualize that the inner surface of the ball is conditionally split into the temporal areas of external events' development, for example, into months. When lighting these areas consistently with the light of your events, you safely normalize the events for the next year. At the same moment keep in mind all the time that we in this method of control of eternal life we perceive ourselves particularly inside of all the phenomena of infinite reality, even if we consider a very short period of time of this eternal life.

Is It Possible to Protect Oneself from Terrorist Attacks in the Subway? Testimonial of Elena Dagunts

I remember such a poll staged in one of the online publications...

Is it really possible?

Because one never knows where one will gain and where one will lose...

Or **"had I known where I would fall, I wouldn't have come to that place at all"** and so on.

However, if you stand on the position of the controller, i.e. the person who voluntarily takes responsibility for everything that happens in his world, or, as St. Seraphim of Sarov says: "Save yourself and around you thousands will be saved", then Yes! – it is possible to avoid any destructive information.

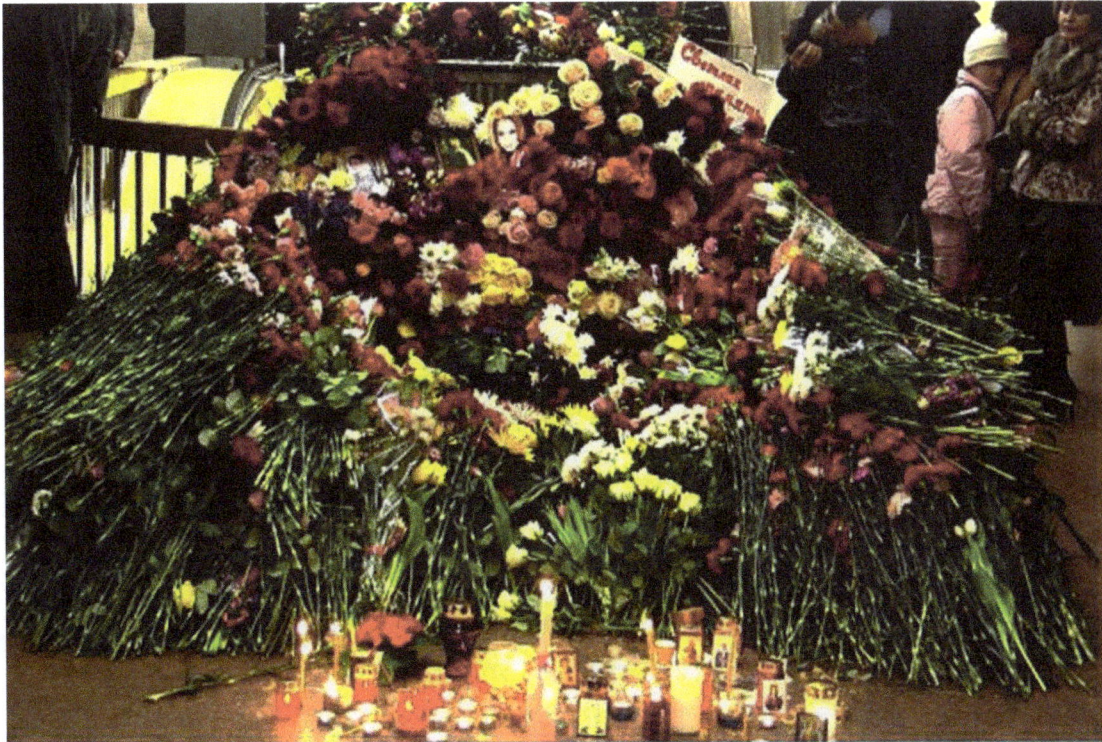

March 29, 2010.
The terrorist attacks in Moscow metro stations
«Lubyanka» and «Park Kultury».

"If people have understood that the problem lies not in machines, but in the information control, exactly in the task and the role of man in the structure of the world, the evolution development would have had a different direction"
Grigori Grabovoi

This is not an unfounded reasoning, but the knowledge, proven in practice.

March 29, 2010 there were 2 explosions in Moscow metro: at the stations "Lubyanka" and "Park Kultury". It was Monday, I went to work and arrived at the station "Park Kultury" at 8:40 am – at time when there was a terrorist attack.

That terrible event made me look at everything, at the way we live, under a different angle of view.

I consider this day my second birthday. People who are far from the Teachings responded to my miraculous rescue with the words: "You were born in a shirt; you're lucky..." But I know that I was saved by controlling technology through own mind that I used in the subway for half an hour before the explosion without a break.

However, let`s go step by step.

First I want to say about my state early in the morning of March 29, 6:30 am – I'm going to work to the University to the 9-hour lecture and I do not understand what is happening to me – everything goes wrong and I do not want to go anywhere. Then I did not connect that my unusual state with some upcoming no-go, just tracked that there was something wrong with me.

At the interchange station "Biblioteka Lenina" about 8:00 am when I got there, there were assembled so many people, another 15 minutes there were no trains. When the train finally arrived, I had to miss it, because it was awfully crowded. All this time, while I stood on the platform waiting for the train, and later, when I managed to take the next train, I worked through my consciousness using the technologies of Grigori Grabovoi. The inner voice did not let me stop for a minute to have a rest. I worked using all methods that were known to me by that time for many times, repeating them again and again.

We were going to the station "Park Cultury" 20 minutes instead of 5 minutes. By that time the explosion on the station "Lubyanka" had already occurred. But the passengers were not told about it. On the radio there announced that for technical reasons, the time between the departures of the trains increased. And people were advised to use ground transport.

I realized that I was very late for classes at the University and continued to work on methods of control of events on the Teachings of Grigori Grabovoi. And I set the aim at the optimization of the events for myself and for the people around me, in order everybody including me arrived at the place of their

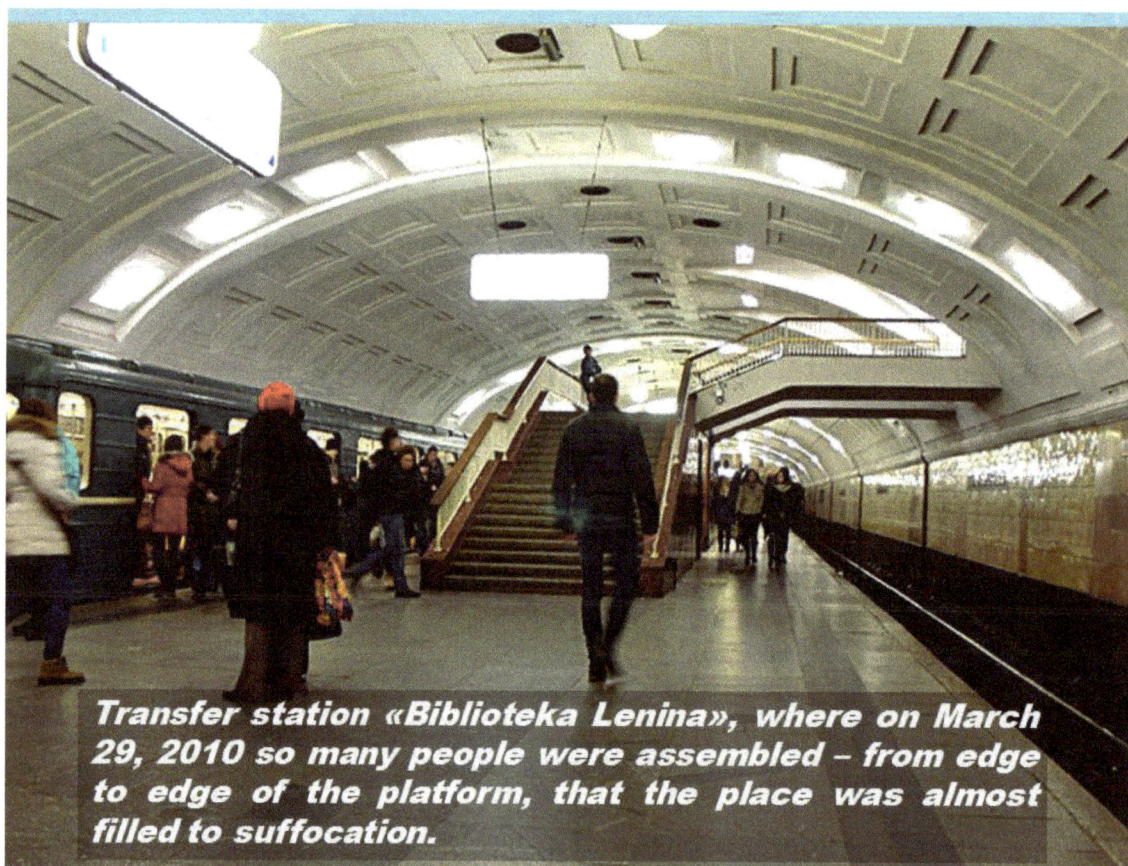

Transfer station «Biblioteka Lenina», where on March 29, 2010 so many people were assembled – from edge to edge of the platform, that the place was almost filled to suffocation.

destination on time and at the elimination of technical problems.

We arrived at the station "Park Cultury" by 8:40 am. And in a moment at the station there occurred an explosion. There were two claps not very loud, but terrible, after them the space immediately changed. Everything was covered with smoke and stench. It became difficult to breath. There lay people on the platform in the distance of around 15 meters from me.

The realization that it had been a terroristic attack came later.

People began heading for the exit of the subway. It was a huge number of people, but nevertheless there was no panic, people helped each other, supported each other, immediately parted and formed a corridor, when from behind somebody asked the way to carry the wounded.

My control worked out as follows:

1. I missed the epicenter of the explosion;

2. people who were in the radius of 10 meters from me – were not injured. That is, those who were next to me – they didn't suffer;

3. what's also important – at «Park Kultury» there was no panic (later from the media I learned that in the «Lubyanka» there was panic and a crush/jam, people suffered from it too). And on the station «Park Kultury» people made way for each other, helped each other, immediately parted and formed a corridor, when from behind somebody asked the way to carry the wounded.

4. from the media I later learned that on the station «Park Kultury» there were killed people and injured people almost 2 times less than on the station «Lubyanka». And the power of explosion was almost 2 times less.

5. So I was only 20 minutes late for the classes. It must be taken into account that I was going to work from unfamiliar place – I had to get out of the subway at the station «Universitet» but because of the explosion I got out of the subway at the station «Park Kultury». Immediately right in front of me the right bus stopped, which was going to the University.

Here I want to also say that no one is immune from falling into some critical situation for different reasons, everyone may have his own ones. But owning those technologies that are brought to the mankind by Grigori Grabovoi, we stay alive, unharmed and in varying degrees, we are able to assist the people who occurred to be next to us.

And this event, terrible event, that happened to me, helped me to realize – what is important in life and what is not.

Before that I was always afraid to be late for work, to violate the established order, that`s why I never used surface transport, though I lived 20 minutes ' drive from the University. Was always afraid in the morning to beat the traffic and went to work by subway using circuitous route.

After this explosion everything in my head as if fell into place. The most important thing in life is to protect life, to save oneself and all the people from the hatred, aggression, fear and violence; to promote love and technology of salvation to all people.

And to come on time to work, say, or pass-take exams – it is secondary, it is not the main thing. This is important, of course, but it is not the main thing.

The main thing now – to save life on our planet, save the people and disseminate the technology of salvation, anti-terrorist technology worldwide.

September 2, 2010; completed in September 2016.

Magic Word – Resurrection

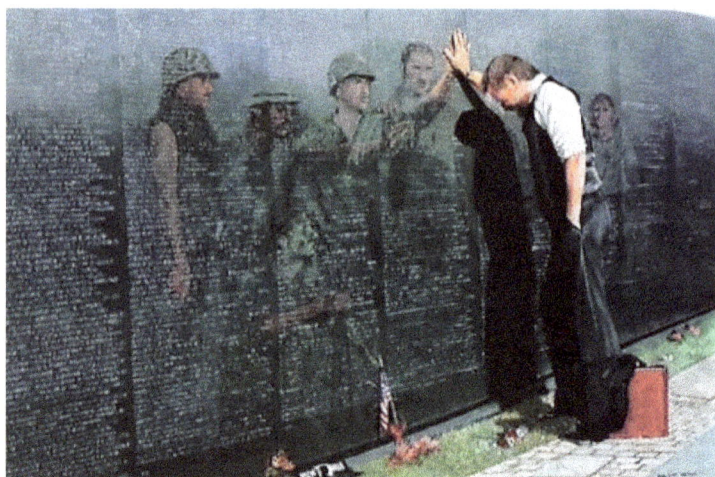

In 2004 – 2005, the word RESURRECTION was absurd, rude and blatantly used by certain media for the introduction of information substitution, that is, terrorism and terrorists in Beslan as if were replaced with the raising of children. The very concept of RESURRECTION, it implies that *"at any changes the principle of non-killing should always remain immutable", "every destruction is pointless because everything can be restored".*

Combining through the name of the city of Beslan different notions of terrorism and RESURRECTION, journalists thereby brought into the Collective Consciousness the structure of misunderstanding of the running events that affected the result of the spiritual development of the country, expressed at the vulnerable part of the population in the negation both restoration technologies and the ability to control events.

Therefore, it is at least silly to listen to the media about Grigori Grabovoi and his Teachings, because the media doesn`t talk about the content of the Teachings, and they do not know it, and use the applied substitution of concepts in any reference to the terrorist attack in Beslan, illegally linking Beslan to the name of the author of the Teachings.

It has been implanted in the mind of people for long moths (and now already – for years), thereby widespread claims of citizens to the errors made during the anti-terrorist operation were withdrawn, and the attention was drawn away, to completely different direction.

And we must give due to the fact that the correct understanding has remained in the city, that is Beslan`s residents themselves have internal understanding, though partly the propaganda of slander touched them, too.

The RESURRECTION has always been present in our life, it has been in our mind from fairy tales since childhood: there we learned about dead water and water of life, which revived the dead, about magical Golden apples, about bathing of the good fellow in boiling water, spring water and boiling milk, which gave the hero beauty and strength. The tales prepared children for the fact that a man was able to control the events, was able to recover his health and youth.

Of course, the word RESURRECTION is the magic word, which according to its vibrations is comparable with the reading of prayers, so anyway it as if works in the right direction towards the restoration of all matter, but

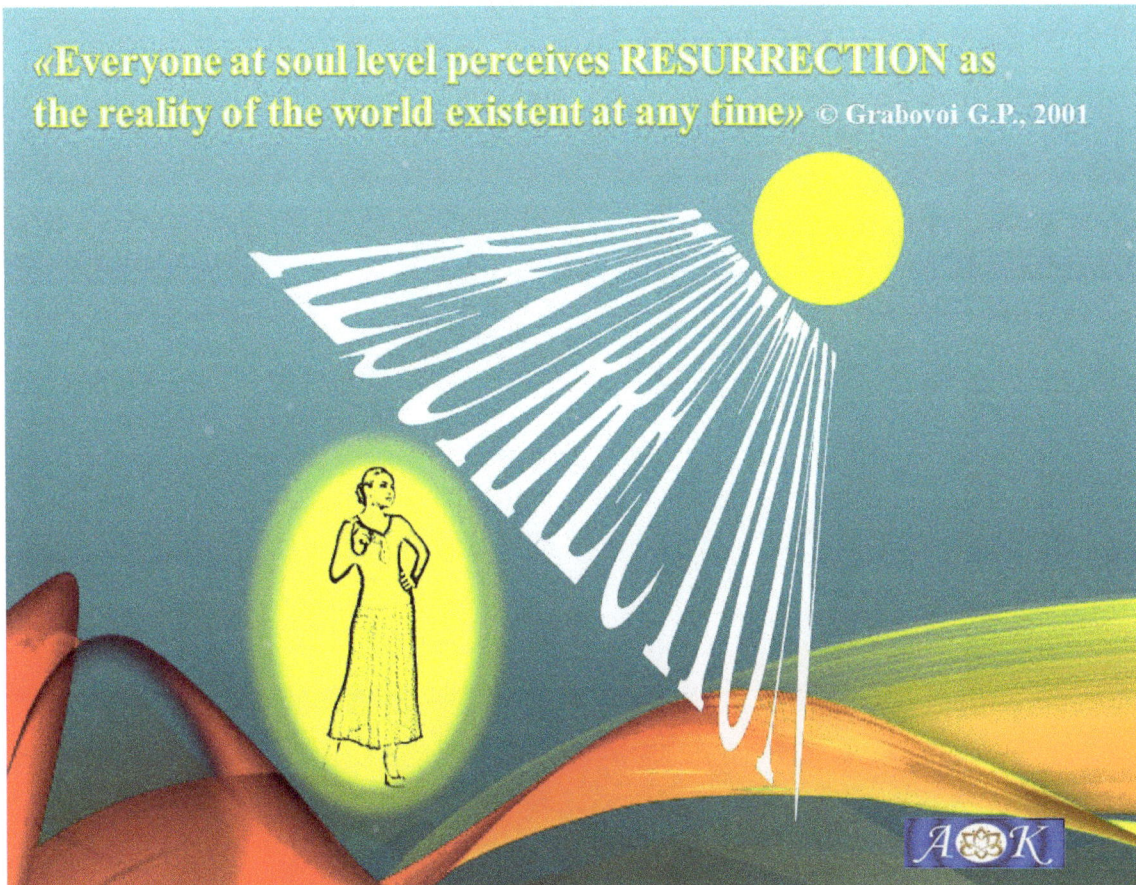

«Everyone at soul level perceives RESURRECTION as the reality of the world existent at any time» © Grabovoi G.P., 2001

nevertheless the people who believe false information, close for themselves the MAGIC of RESURRECTION.

So, about RESURRECTION from the Teachings of Grigori Petrovich Grabovoi, from his book **"Resurrection of people and eternal life from now on is our reality!"**.

1. *"For many people RESURRECTION is something symbolic, though everyone at soul level perceives RESURRECTION as the reality of the World existent at any time"*

2. *"...from a certain perspective RESURRECTION is a standard procedure, which expands the state of consciousness to the level when coming back to life is possible. And that's precisely why RESURRECTION can be taught, just as any other standard procedure can".*

3. *"RESURRECTION is in fact the control of the entire external space".*

4. *"...by visualizing a body, one can transmit the knowledge of RESURRECTION to its soul"*.

5. *"... at present RESURRECTION is still perceived by many as a miracle; because there are still people, who have no genuine understanding of the fact that in actuality RESURRECTION is a standard procedure, and soon RESURRECTION will be in the nature of things, it will become a norm of life"*.

6. *And in the not distant future, when at least a part of society will realize, that the process of RESURRECTION is a normal standard procedure, RESURRECTION will be occurring faster due to society's readiness to accept this phenomenon"*.

In fact, the RESURRECTION is not already magic in the truest sense of the word, because nowadays it is becoming a reality, thanks to the technologies that are increasingly used by people practicing the Teachings of Grigori Grabovoi.

September 18, 2016.

List of the translations

Translated by Elena Dagunts:

1. Recovery of computer control system;
2. Oxygen increasing in the room according to the Teachings of Grigori Grabovoi;
3. Rejuvenation for women and men;
4. Rejuvenating through the novelty of perception and a photo;
5. Work with an aggressive person using the number series 14789;
6. The normalization of the reception of information – of any block that you build;
7. Recovery impulse from palms of child;
8. The technology of the gold ball. You need to find a way;
9. Snowball;
10. Magic word – RESURRECTION.

Translated by Irina Mokrushina:

1. Level of Beauty and Eternity of the Teaching of Grigori Grabovoi;
2. Technology of rejuvenating by the book of Grigori Grabovoi "Number series of psychological normalization";
3. Direct access to the event structure to restore health;
4. Remove negative information from events;
5. How the world speaks with us;
6. How to help those people who have lost;
7. The "eights" nearby the sofa or exit from control;
8. To find a lost thing is a manifested result;

List of references

1. Грабовой Г.П. «Иррациональные методы предотвращения глобальных катастрофических процессов, представляющих угрозу всему миру», © Грабовой Г.П., 2001;
2. Грабовой Г.П. «Технология спасения и гармоничного развития. Методы управления посредством звука и форм», © Грабовой Г.П., 2002;
3. Грабовой Г.П. «Учение Григория Грабового О Боге. Частное управление через общую область информации», © Грабовой Г.П., 2005;
4. Grabovoi G.P. "Number Series of Psychological Normalization", 2003;
5. Grabovoi G.P. "Manifestations of Eternity" (volume 1);

6. Грабовой Г.П. "Учение Григория Грабового о Боге. Методы Вечной Жизни", © Грабовой Г.П., 2005;

7. Грабовой Г.П. "Учение Григория Грабового о Боге. Создание структуры Вечности", © Грабовой Г.П., 2005;

8. Grabovoi G.P. "The unified system of knowledge", © Grabovoi G.P., 1996;

9. Грабовой Г.П. "Учение Григория Грабового о Боге. Управленческие системы будущего", © Грабовой Г.П., 2005;

10. Grabovoi G.P. "Hayrúkulus", 2000;

11. Interview of G.P. Grabovoi to the magazine "SOBESEDNIK" of October 4, 2005.

12. Grabovoi G.P. "Technology of transfer of the result received from control in one area of own Consciousness to another one to prevent global catastrophes", © Grabovoi G.P., 2001;

13. Грабовой Г.П. «Управление управляющим импульсом», © Грабовой Г.П., 2005;

14. Грабовой Г.П. «Методы управления посредством своего Сознания, основанные на структуре восприятия для регулировки системы предотвращения макрокатастроф и прямого доступа в структуру события», © Грабовой Г.П., 2002;

15. Grabovoi G.P. "The beginning of the educational program on Grigori Grabovoi`s Teachings";

16. Грабовой Г.П. «Учение Григория Грабового о Боге. Действие вечной реальности», © Грабовой Г.П., 2004;

17. Грабовой Г.П. «Учение Григория Грабового о Боге. Система предотвращения терроризма», © Грабовой Г.П., 2004;

18. Грабовой Г.П. «Учение Григория Грабового о Боге. Практика межтерриториального управления», © Грабовой Г.П., 2006;

19. Grabovoi G.P. "Teaching of Grigori Grabovoi about God. Technologies of development of memory for eternal life", © Grabovoi G.P., 2015;

20. The webinar of Grigori Grabovoi "Teaching of Grigori Grabovoi about God. Methods of control the eternal life" given on October 13, 2015;

21. Грабовой Г.П. «Учение Григория Грабового о Боге. Динамическая структуризация Души», © Грабовой Г.П., 2004;

22. Elena Dagunts "Is it possible to protect oneself from terrorist attacks in the subway?"

23. Grabovoi G.P. "The Resurrection of People and Eternal Life from Now on Is Our Reality!", © Grabovoi G.P., 2001.

www.ingramcontent.com/pod-product-compliance
Lightning Source LLC
Chambersburg PA
CBHW050936210326
41518CB00023BB/2598

* 9 7 8 3 9 4 5 5 4 9 3 6 0 *